Psychological Treatment of

Cardiac Patients

Clinical Health Psychology Series

Psychological Treatment of Cardiac Patients
Matthew M. Burg

Psychological Treatment of Medical Patients in Integrated Primary Care
Anne C. Dobmeyer

Psychological Treatment of Patients With Cancer
Ellen A. Dornelas

Psychological Treatment of **Cardiac Patients**

MATTHEW M. BURG

CLINICAL HEALTH PSYCHOLOGY SERIES

ELLEN A. DORNELAS, Series Editor

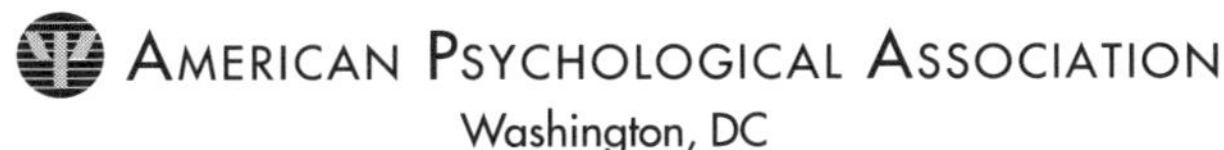
American Psychological Association
Washington, DC

Published by
American Psychological Association
750 First Street, NE
Washington, DC 20002
www.apa.org

APA Order Department
P.O. Box 92984
Washington, DC 20090-2984
Phone: (800) 374-2721; Direct: (202) 336-5510
Fax: (202) 336-5502; TDD/TTY: (202) 336-6123
Online: http://www.apa.org/pubs/books
E-mail: order@apa.org

In the U.K., Europe, Africa, and the Middle East, copies may be ordered from
Eurospan Group
c/o Pegasus Drive
Stratton Business Park
Biggleswade Bedfordshire
SG18 8TQ United Kingdom
Phone: +44 (0) 1767 604972
Fax: +44 (0) 1767 601640
Online: https://www.eurospanbookstore.com/apa
E-mail: eurospan@turpin-distribution.com

Typeset in Minion by Circle Graphics, Inc., Columbia, MD

Printer: Edwards Brothers Malloy, Lillington, NC
Cover Designer: Mercury Publishing Services, Inc., Rockville, MD

Library of Congress Cataloging-in-Publication Data

Names: Burg, Matthew M., author.
Title: Psychological treatment of cardiac patients / Matthew M. Burg.
Description: First edition. | Washington, DC : American Psychological Association, [2018] | Series: Clinical health psychology book series | Includes bibliographical references and index.
Identifiers: LCCN 2017027818 | ISBN 9781433828294 | ISBN 1433828294
Subjects: LCSH: Coronary heart disease—Psychological aspects.
Classification: LCC RC685.C6 B88 2018 | DDC 616.1/230651—dc23 LC record available at https://lccn.loc.gov/2017027818

British Library Cataloguing-in-Publication Data
A CIP record is available from the British Library.

Printed in the United States of America
First Edition

http://dx.doi.org/10.1037/0000070-000

10 9 8 7 6 5 4 3 2 1

Contents

Series Foreword

Mental health practitioners working in medicine represent the vanguard of psychological practice. As scientific discovery and advancement in medicine has rapidly evolved in recent decades, it has been a challenge for clinical health psychology practice to keep pace.

In a fast-changing field, and with a paucity of practice-based research, classroom models of health psychology practice often do not translate well to clinical care. All too often, health psychologists work in silos, with little appreciation of how advancement in one area might inform another. The goal of the Clinical Health Psychology Series is to change these trends and provide a comprehensive yet concise overview of the essential elements of clinical practice in specific areas of health care. The future of 21st-century health psychology depends on the ability of new practitioners to be innovative and to generalize their knowledge across domains. To this end, the series will focus on a variety of topics and provide both a foundation as well as specific clinical examples for mental health professionals who are new to the field.

Working with Susan Reynolds, senior acquisitions editor at the American Psychological Association (APA Books), I am proud to have had an opportunity to edit this book series. We have chosen authors who are recognized experts in the field and who are rethinking the practice of health psychology to be aligned with modern drivers of health care such as population health, cost of care, quality of care, and customer experience.

Dr. Mathew Burg's book *Psychological Treatment of Cardiac Patients* draws on his vast experience as one of the pioneers in the field of cardiac psychology. His pragmatic approach to psychological assessment and intervention will be invaluable to mental health practitioners, helping them negotiate the challenges inherent in treating a patient population with considerable variation in the manifestation of their disease. This book provides an in-depth review of the anatomy, physiology, and medical approaches to diagnosing and treating heart disease. Dr. Burg tackles topics that have often received little attention in this field, such as sleep dysregulation, sexual dysfunction, and end-of-life care. *Psychological Treatment of Cardiac Patients* will also be informative for students seeking to practice in clinical health psychology, as well as for experienced therapists seeking greater understanding of their clientele who have heart disease.

It is rare to find books from experienced health psychology researchers aimed at the clinical audience. Yet it is only through this type of cross-pollination that the field of cardiac psychology can undergo the reengineering necessary to drive the science forward and speed the dissemination of evidence-based practices. Thus, I am tremendously indebted to Dr. Burg for his commitment to the field and contribution of this important work.

—Ellen A. Dornelas, PhD
Series Editor

Acknowledgments

The field of cardiovascular behavioral medicine—or cardiac psychology—has received a great deal of attention because of groundbreaking research by two cardiologists, Meyer Friedman and Ray Roseman. This book is indebted to their earlier work on "behavior pattern A," and also to Dr. Ellen Dornelas and her 2008 book, *Psychotherapy With Cardiac Patients: Behavioral Cardiology in Practice.*

Psychological Treatment of
Cardiac Patients

Introduction

Coronary heart disease (CHD), which broadly comprises the full range of disease that strikes the heart, is the leading cause of death and disability in the United States. According to Mozaffarian et al. (2016), over 28 million U.S. adults are diagnosed with heart disease, and each year over half a million people have a first heart attack, with another 300,000 experiencing a second such event. Each year approximately 610,000 people in the United States die of heart disease, representing a quarter of all deaths annually. This disease is more likely to strike men than women, and the risk is considerably higher for non-Hispanic Black males and Black females than for their White counterparts. The last decade saw an almost 30% decline in death attributable to CHD, but in 2013 CHD still accounted for almost one third of all deaths, making it the number one killer. CHD is typically thought of as a disease of aging, yet over 10% of individuals

http://dx.doi.org/10.1037/0000070-001
Psychological Treatment of Cardiac Patients, by M. M. Burg

between the ages of 45 and 65 have heart disease, and approximately one quarter of Americans who die of this disease are less than 65 years of age. Furthermore, over a third of these deaths occur before the age of 75, an age younger than the average life expectancy in the United States today. Each year approximately 360,000 Americans experience out-of-hospital catastrophic cardiac arrhythmic events or cardiac arrest, and little more than 10% of these individuals survive to hospital discharge.

There are more than 17 million individuals living in the United States with chronic CHD and many million more with hypertension, cerebrovascular disease (stroke), and peripheral vascular disease. Heart failure (HF) is another clinical presentation of CHD and occurs when the heart muscle does not pump blood as well as it should or once did because the muscle is too weak or stiff to fill and pump efficiently. In 2013, one in nine death certificates in the United States included HF. The number of any-mention deaths attributable to HF has not appreciably changed over the past 2 decades (approximately 285,000 annually). In addition, hospital discharges for HF have remained stable, with first-listed discharges of over one million annually (statistics reported by Mozaffarian et al., 2016).

It should be apparent that CHD has profound costs to the public health, and this remains true despite the revolution in CHD-related care that has occurred over the past 2 decades. Approximately 40% of the chronic disease burden is attributed to lifestyle and mental health factors, indicating the profound potential for psychological and psychosocial interventions to reduce CHD incidence (Mozaffarian et al., 2016). Indeed, efforts to reduce the risk of first cardiac events—for example, through efforts such as smoking cessation and increased physical activity—have been part of the success that has been realized in recent years. In addition to the contributions that psychosocial and lifestyle factors have made to the onset of disease is the role these factors play for patients after a first cardiac event. For example, patients are faced with many lifestyle adjustments after a cardiac event, and many patients additionally experience a profound psychological disruption to their sense of personal integrity. There are stresses that can accompany the medical treatments needed for heart disease, some more acute—such as angioplasty—and some lifelong—such as medication regimens. Although a period of psychological adjustment (e.g., feelings of anxiety and depression) after a heart attack can be expected, longer lasting and frank depression, whether at a level sufficient for diagnosis or a "subsyndromal" level, not only affects quality of life but also contributes to recurrent cardiac events and early mortality. Thus, the role of the psychologist can be important not only in the prevention of CHD but also in the treatment of the patient after a cardiac event.

This book is an introduction to and a primer for the clinical practice of cardiovascular behavioral medicine and behavioral cardiology and is appropriate for advanced students and mental health professionals who are new to this specialty. Throughout this book, clinical examples are used to illustrate the disease presentation, subsequent treatments, and the psychosocial issues that both contribute to heart disease and are sequelae to cardiac events.

The book is not intended as sufficient to inform practice in the cardiologic "space." The psychologist without specific advanced training in this area can use this text to gain a basic understanding, but it is essential that he or she pursue advanced training before initiating practice in this area. Failure to do so may place the psychologist at risk of violating the Ethical Standards in the American Psychological Association (2017a) *Ethical Principles of Psychologists and Code of Conduct* concerning practice competence. This volume does not include an exhaustive review of all literature relevant to the field but instead provides an overview and introduction to this evolving area of clinical practice. Areas not discussed in greater detail include heart diseases that affect children and young adults and genetic-based diseases such as those involving conduction disorders. Nor is more detail provided about the emerging understanding of posttraumatic stress disorder as a factor influencing cardiac outcomes. However, this book does provide a foundation of knowledge and understanding for the pursuit of more detailed knowledge, understanding, and skill with proper supervision and guidance.

Part I of this book is devoted to a detailed overview of the heart—its structure and function, the processes involved in the regulation of the heart and associated processes and organ systems, and the factors that contribute to heart disease onset and prognosis. In this overview, disease conditions that affect the heart are described, providing the health psychologist with the depth of knowledge requisite for interacting knowledgeably with cardiac patients and the full range of health care providers involved in their care. I devote particular emphasis to the processes by which CHD develops and cardiac events are triggered and to the pathways understood to link psychological factors to CHD. Whereas Chapter 1 is devoted to cardiac anatomy and function, Chapter 2 delves most specifically into disease etiology, while also providing a historical perspective on cardiovascular behavioral medicine and cardiac psychology. The etiological and sociocultural context serves to identify issues related to vulnerable subgroups. This section of the book culminates with Chapter 3, which provides an overview of the standard and emerging medical treatments that are available to patients, with a description of the various psychological issues these treatments may produce.

Part II focuses on psychological assessment and treatment of patients with CHD. Chapter 4 is devoted to depression, a condition that occurs for up to one quarter of patients after a cardiac event and that, if persistent, contributes to recurrent cardiac events and early mortality. I review the pathways thought to link depression to these events, as well as methods used to assess depression in this population and the clinical trials literature concerning depression treatments for patients with heart disease. I also review the current status of recommendations for addressing depression in patients with heart disease and the integration of depression care with overall cardiologic care.

Anxiety in patients with heart disease is the subject of Chapter 5. Like the chapter on depression, this chapter focuses on etiology, behavioral factors, pathways linking anxiety to cardiac-related outcomes, and methods used for assessment and treatment. The focus on assessment also includes assessment of anxiety for patients with specific cardiac conditions, particularly those whose condition requires treatment with an implantable cardioverter defibrillator. I discuss issues of comorbidity with depression, common for both cardiac patients and the general population, as well as issues related to gender, such as the higher incidence of anxiety disorders in women.

Sleep and sleep dysregulation are common in cardiac patients and often part of the etiology underlying heart disease development and expression. In Chapter 6, I provide an overview of sleep, along with a review of sleep disorders and the role of sleep in heart disease. I also discuss methods used to assess sleep, including emerging wrist-worn technologies that assess sleep quality more objectively than is possible with self-report. In addition, I provide a more detailed description of standard sleep disorder treatment—for example, improving sleep hygiene and using cognitive behavioral therapy for insomnia. The chapter also includes a discussion of sleep apnea, which is particularly common among patients with HF.

Sexual functioning is often negatively affected by cardiac events, in large part due to the anxiety that accompanies return to previous activities and the side effects that accompany cardiac medications for some patients. Chapter 7 discusses methods used to assess sexual issues and functioning in cardiac patients, with a more focused discussion of specific assessment tools for men and women. I discuss approaches to treatment and the outstanding questions regarding best approaches, particularly for women with heart disease.

Chapter 8 focuses on social support and the effects of heart disease in the context of the family. I describe the different types of social support—structural, functional, and so forth—and the research linking social support to heart disease. I also discuss the research concerning social support interventions for cardiac patients and make recommendations for how the health psychologist practicing in the cardiology space might proceed.

Chapter 9 is devoted to end-of-life issues in cardiac care. This chapter, in particular, serves as a context for discussing HF, which represents the progression of heart disease to a terminal state. I discuss the treatment of HF through the use of devices—implanted defibrillators, ventricular assist devices—and the emergence of a palliative care model for the treatment of advanced disease and for addressing end-of-life issues.

Part III concludes the book with Chapter 10, which concerns the integration of psychological and medical aspects of care for patients with heart disease. Although this is an underlying theme for each of the chapters, the absence of a psychologist or other mental health provider from cardiologic care teams as a given throughout the United States remains a point of consternation and, in the view of this writer, an important obstacle to the reduction in heart disease incidence and the burden and suffering associated with heart disease for the patient and his or her family members. In this final chapter, I discuss the issues involved in this state of affairs and present ideas for addressing them.

ONE

OVERVIEW OF HEART DISEASE FOR THE MENTAL HEALTH PROFESSIONAL

1

An Overview of Heart Disease for the Mental Health Professional

The heart is at once a simple and complex organ, with many features involved in both its normal and diseased function. The base of knowledge regarding its structure and its function is rich. Although a detailed understanding of how the heart and the cardiovascular system work may not be a typical component of training for the psychologist, a conversant understanding is essential for the psychologist who practices in cardiovascular behavioral medicine or cardiac psychology. This level of understanding will ensure that he or she can interact with cardiologists and nurses as a peer and can interact knowledgeably with often highly informed patients and family members, while also more completely appreciating the experiences of these individuals. A great deal of anatomical information is presented in this chapter, and readers are referred to Figures 1.1, 1.2, and 1.3 to guide them through the descriptions.

http://dx.doi.org/10.1037/0000070-002
Psychological Treatment of Cardiac Patients, by M. M. Burg

THE HEART AND VENTRICLES

The heart is a muscle shaped like a cone (see Figure 1.1). It works as a pump by contracting, with each contraction pumping blood to the lungs, where the blood gives up waste gases and is reoxygenated. From the lungs, that blood returns to the heart to be pumped to the rest of the body, returning to again be pumped to the lungs, and so on. The heart is made up of four muscular chambers, defined by side—left and right—and function—upper chambers, or *atria*, and lower chambers, or *ventricles*. The atria are chambers that receive returning blood—the right atrium from the body, the left atrium from the lungs—and the ventricles are chambers from which the blood is pumped—the right ventricle to the lungs, the left ventricle to the body. Thus, the right side of the heart is where the blood returns to after coursing through the body and from where it is pumped to the lungs, and the left side is where the blood returns to after being oxygenated by the lungs and from where the blood is pumped to the body. The left ventricle does a great deal more work than the right and, indeed, the overall health of the left ventricle—measured as the percentage of blood pumped out of the chamber with each contraction, an index called the *left ventricular ejection fraction*—is among the most significant determinants of outcomes for patients with coronary heart disease (CHD). Although the heart does its work by contracting, that contraction is not a single "spasm" involving the contraction of each chamber, but rather a two-stage process that can be heard as the "lub-dub" of a single heartbeat, the atria contracting first to move blood to the ventricles, the ventricles contracting next to move blood to the lungs and body.

THE HEART VALVES

The smooth and efficient movement of blood requires valves so as to ensure that with the contraction of each chamber the blood can only move in the required direction, rather than back into the chamber. Four major valves in the heart direct blood flow forward and prevent backward leakage. Thus, on the right side, the *tricuspid valve* is between the right atrium

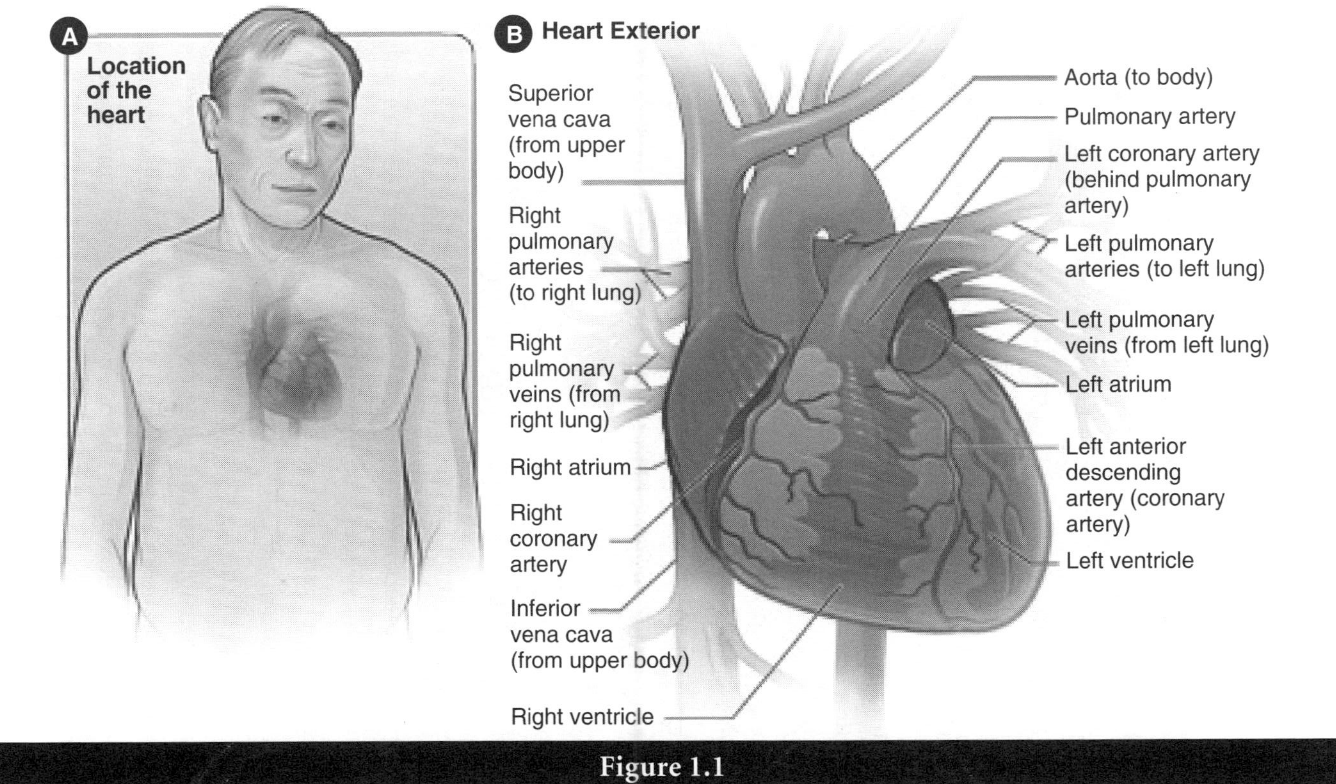

Figure 1.1

Exterior anatomy of the heart, showing the atria and ventricles, the major arteries and veins leaving and returning to the heart, and the coronary arteries. From "Anatomy of the Heart," by National Institutes of Health, U.S. Department of Health and Human Services, 2011 (https://www.nhlbi.nih.gov/health/health-topics/topics/hhw/anatomy). In the public domain.

and right ventricle, and the *pulmonic valve* is between the right ventricle and pulmonary artery through which blood is sent to the lungs; on the left side, the *mitral valve* is between the left atrium and left ventricle, and the *aortic valve* is between the left ventricle and the *aorta*, the largest artery, through which blood is sent throughout the body (see Figure 1.2).

The valves are composed of a base and either two or three leaflets (depending on the valve) that open and close. Papillary muscles and the chordae tendineae that project from them attach at the edges of tricuspid and mitral valve leaflets, whereas the base of the valves is attached to fibrous rings that anchor the valve between the heart chambers. This arrangement allows for the valves to open under pressure from the contracting heart chamber (e.g., left atrium) on one side, while returning to their closed formation when the next chamber (e.g., left ventricle) contracts. The aortic and pulmonic valves have a similar seating arrangement but do not require the muscular and tendon support for their leaflets to close properly. The valves on the left side can be thought of as the most important valves in the heart, again because of the greater work done by the left side of the heart and, given the distance that blood travels, the greater pumping force or pressures involved.

THE ELECTRICAL, OR CONDUCTION, SYSTEM

What of the process that controls the pumping action of the heart? Contraction is an electromechanical process that is regulated by an impulse conducting system. This system is composed of specialized cells that initiate the heartbeat and electrically coordinate the contractions of the atria and ventricles. The *sinoatrial* (SA) *node* is a small mass of fibers located in the wall at the top of the right atrium. It is the natural pacemaker of the heart and is responsible for initiating the cardiac cycle or heartbeat. It spontaneously generates an electrical impulse, which is then conducted electrically throughout the heart. The SA node is richly innervated by the two branches of the autonomic nervous system (ANS), with both parasympathetic nervous system (PNS) and sympathetic nervous system (SNS) fibers. This anatomic arrangement leaves the SA node subject to

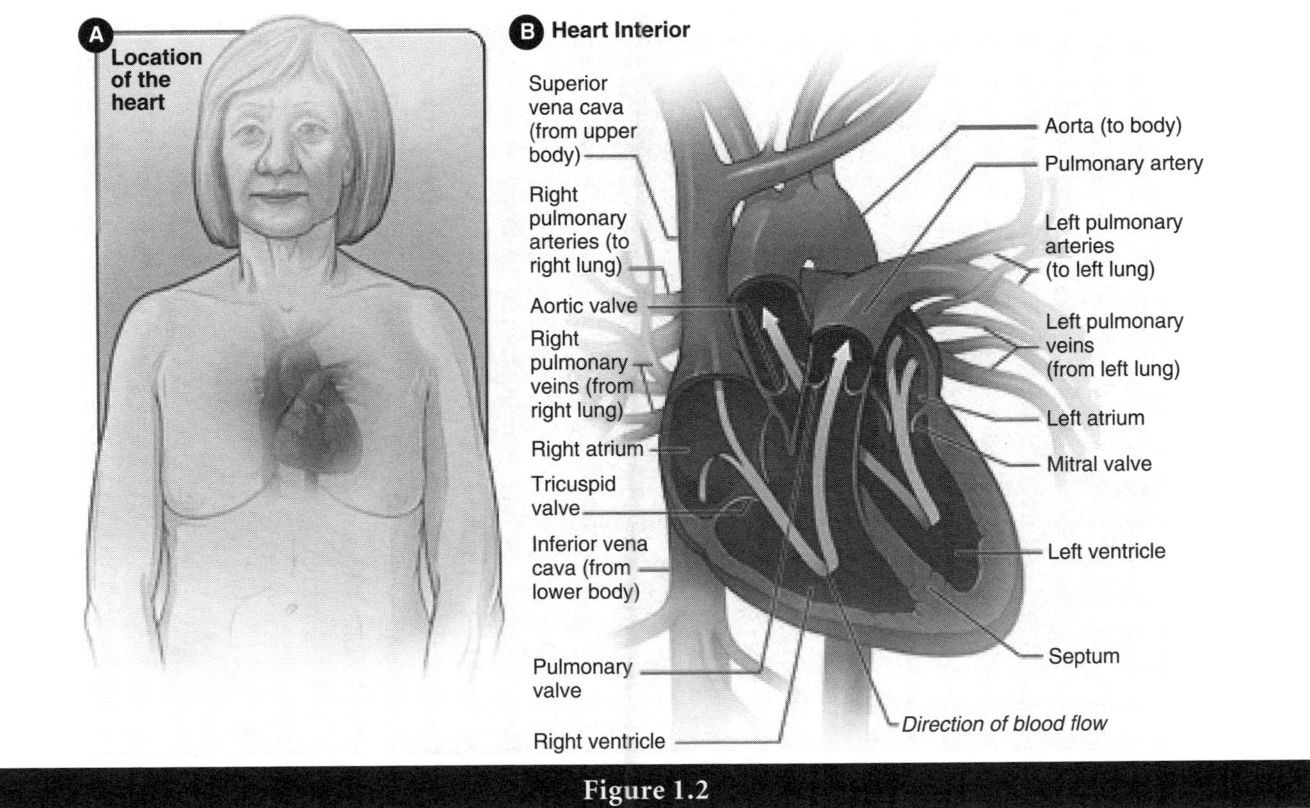

Figure 1.2

Interior anatomy of the heart, showing the heart chambers and valves and great vessels, and depicting the flow of blood through the heart. From "Anatomy of the Heart," by National Institutes of Health, U.S. Department of Health and Human Services, 2011 (https://www.nhlbi.nih.gov/health/health-topics/topics/hhw/anatomy). In the public domain.

paired and opposed autonomic influences that can speed up or slow down the firing rate.

The *atrioventricular* (AV) *node* is the next component of the cardiac conduction system, located at the bottom of the right atrium. The AV node descends in the heart, becoming the *bundle of His*,[1] which perforates the *interventricular septum* (the muscle wall separating the left and right ventricles) and bifurcates into two "bundle branches" (right and left). These two bundle branches further descend in the septum, with each further branching to innervate the ventricles.

The cardiac conduction system coordinates the mechanical activity of the muscle cells—*myocytes*—of the heart. A wave of electrical discharge spreads out from the SA node. This both provokes the contraction of the myocytes in the atria and activates the AV node. The AV node delays impulses by approximately 0.12 seconds, a delay in the cardiac pulse that ensures that the myocytes of the atria have contracted and the atria have ejected their blood into the ventricles before the electrical impulses of the AV node cause the myocytes of the ventricles to contract. In essence, this ensures that the ventricles are full of blood before contracting, thereby providing for the efficient movement of blood from atria, to ventricles, and out of the heart.

At rest, the *sinus rate*—or rate of firing by the SA node—is mostly influenced by *vagal tone*—by the PNS—whereas under demand conditions, such as with physical exertion or psychological stress, the rate is under greater input by the SNS through adrenergic (i.e., involving adrenaline) stimulation. Stimulation through the PNS *vagus nerves* causes a decrease in the SA node firing rate and thereby a decrease in the heart rate, whereas stimulation via SNS fibers causes an increase in the SA node firing rate and thereby an increase in both the heart rate and force of ventricular contraction. SNS fibers can increase the force of contraction because, in addition to innervating the SA and AV nodes, they innervate the atria and ventricles themselves.

[1] The bundle of His is named after Wilhelm His Jr., a Swiss cardiologist who discovered it in 1893.

THE AORTA

The aorta is the first major distribution point for pumped blood. It is shaped like an inverted *U*, with a first short ascending section followed by a long descending section. The first two branches of the aorta are the *coronary arteries*, left and right, which provide blood to the heart muscle itself, perfusing the heart and providing the oxygen and nutrients required for the heart to do its pumping work. These are relatively small branches, and their "takeoff" is just outside the aortic valve and adjacent to the aortic valve leaflets. The next branches on the ascending section are large, and these deliver blood to the head, neck, and arms. The next branches are on the descending *thoracic aorta*, which travels down through the chest, with small branches supplying blood to the ribs and other chest structures, and the *abdominal aorta* beginning at the diaphragm, splitting to become the paired iliac arteries in the lower abdomen, and then further splitting to deliver blood to the major organs and lower limbs.

CORONARY CIRCULATION

As described earlier, the myocytes of the heart are perfused—provided with oxygen and nutrients—by the right and left coronary arteries; these arise from the root of the aorta, taking off just above the cusps of the aortic valve. The large *left main coronary artery* (LM) quickly divides into the *left anterior descending coronary artery* (LAD) and the *left circumflex coronary artery* (LCx). The LAD descends along the front of the heart, giving off septal and diagonal branches that cover a great deal of the left ventricle and thereby provide the greatest amount of blood supply to that most important chamber. Hence the term *widow maker* to describe major blockages in the upper part of the LAD before the branching occurs—an acute closure of this vessel in the context of an evolving myocardial infarction can be the first sign of underlying CHD in a young man and is often fatal. The LCx passes around to the posterior, or back of the heart, giving off branches called *marginals* that supply the lateral and posterior walls of the left ventricle.

The right coronary artery (RCA) travels along the groove between the posterior right atrium and ventricle, providing blood to the right ventricle. Further branching, the posterior descending artery travels to the apex of the heart (the bottom) and supplies blood to the inferior and posterior walls of the ventricles. Collateral connections of microscopic diameter are found between the coronary arteries. Although these are not visible in the normal heart, they typically become larger when obstructions occur in the main coronary arteries, thereby providing blood flow to portions of the vessel distal from, or beyond, the obstruction.

From their surface or *epicardial* locations, the coronary arteries send perforating arterial projections into the ventricular muscle, forming a richly branching vasculature in the wall of the four heart chambers. This vasculature becomes increasingly smaller in diameter, from epicardial vessels to prearterioles to smaller and smaller arterioles. Finally, from this branching arises a massively dense network of capillaries, the *coronary microvascular bed*, that forms an elaborate network around each cardiac myocyte. This capillary bed perfuses the myocytes and supports proper cellular contraction and, thus, heart function.

Like arteries throughout the body, the coronary arteries are composed of sequential cellular layers, among the most important of which is the *vascular endothelium*. The vascular endothelium is a single layer of cells that lines the lumen of all blood vessels, maintaining vascular homeostasis by releasing bioactive substances to affect vascular tone. *Endothelial dysfunction* is the failure of the endothelium to maintain vascular homeostasis in response to appropriate stimulation. Endothelial dysfunction can be observed even in people without standard risk factors and is accepted as the earliest indicator of a vascular disease process. It is highly predictive of incident CHD events and widely recognized as an independent marker of high CHD risk prior to the clinical manifestation of disease. When CVD risk reduction efforts are mounted, normalization of endothelial function can be observed, thereby providing an early indicator of the success of these efforts in reducing CHD risk.

Physical, metabolic, and neural factors modulate blood flow in the coronary microvascular bed. In the absence of obstructive stenosis (narrowing), the epicardial coronary arteries—the LM, LAD, LCx, RCA, and their main branches—offer little resistance to coronary blood flow and serve mainly as conduit vessels. The coronary microvascular bed mainly functions in a capacitance role, holding 90% of the total myocardial blood volume. Coronary vascular resistance is primarily controlled by the prearterioles (vessels of 500μm in diameter) and arterioles (200μm in diameter). The prearterioles dilate and contract in response to changes in shear stress (a consequence of the movement of blood along the wall of the prearterioles) and intravascular pressure, thereby preserving adequate perfusion pressure distally (or further along the circulatory route). The arterioles are the true regulatory component of coronary circulation, representing the largest proportion of the total coronary vascular resistance.

Arterioles receive ANS innervation and respond to various circulating hormones that regulate their diameter. Endothelium-dependent vasoreactivity prevails in the larger arterioles (100–200μm in diameter) and translates flow-related stimuli into vasomotor responses: vasodilation with a subsequent increase in flow and vasoconstriction with a subsequent decrease in flow. This endothelium-dependent vasoreactivity is to the greatest extent a function of nitric oxide (NO) bioavailability, with the vasodilatory effects of NO counterbalanced by the vasoconstrictive effect of endothelin-1.

Medium-sized microvessels (40–100μm in diameter) react predominantly to intraluminal pressure changes sensed by stretch receptors located in vascular smooth muscle cells; that is, they constrict when the intraluminal pressure increases and, conversely, dilate when the pressure decreases. Finally, the tone of the smaller arterioles is modulated by the metabolic activity of the myocardium. As such, an increase in metabolic activity requires the heart to work more and leads to vasodilatation of the smaller arterioles, which reduces pressure in the medium-sized microvessels, and myogenic dilation (i.e., dilation in the vessel mediated by smooth muscle cells). This, in turn, increases flow upstream, resulting in endothelium-dependent vasodilation. These mechanisms effectively and efficiently allow the microcirculation to regulate myocardial perfusion both at rest and at different levels of myocardial metabolic demand.

THE STRESS RESPONSE AND CARDIOVASCULAR PSYCHOPHYSIOLOGY

The metabolic needs of the body organs are always changing; therefore, regulation of the heart and the overall cardiovascular system must allow for rapid adaptation to address these needs. This regulation includes processes that ensure sufficient systemic and local perfusion pressures as blood is pumped by the heart through the vascular system to the various organs and the lungs. The rate, force, and timing of myocardial contraction are determined by self-regulatory elements, direct neural inputs from the ANS, and ancillary circulatory elements from the ANS and associated pathways, which together determine cardiac output (CO). CO, in turn, is determined by the *stroke volume* (SV)—the volume of blood ejected by the left ventricle during systole (contraction)—and the heart rate, measured in beats per minute. SV is determined both by the amount of blood filling the ventricle during diastole (relaxation between contractions) and by the resistance in the circulation to the contracting ventricle (afterload). Each of these factors varies according to moment-to-moment tissue needs and ANS tone. SNS stimulation can increase the heart rate (contractions per minute), the speed of individual ventricular contractions, and the force of these contractions (e.g., shorter systolic and diastolic intervals, more forceful ejection). Conversely, PNS input can immediately slow heart rate.

Physical exertion illustrates the heart at work. Exertion increases the metabolic requirements of the muscles involved (e.g., the large muscles of the leg during an exercise treadmill test). CO increases through a rise in both heart rate and SV, though the increase in heart rate is greater, from 60 to 160 beats per minute, or about 150%, than that of SV—only 20% of the resting value. Changes in vasculature also affect the heart. At the onset of exertion, metabolic products from the exercising muscles provoke an immediate dilation of the local resistance vessels. The systolic pressure also increases, though diastolic pressure undergoes little change, because of the dilation in the large muscles provoked by local metabolic reflexes.

The stress response to cognitive and emotional, or overall psychologically perceived demands, is different. A fight-or-flight response is initiated in the amygdala, which communicates with the hypothalamus, which in turn communicates with the pituitary gland, prompting the secretion of adrenocorticotropic hormone, in turn prompting the release of cortisol from the adrenal glands (the hypothalamic–pituitary–adrenal cortex axis). The adrenals more quickly release epinephrine into the circulation. The initial response and subsequent reactions are triggered in an effort to create a boost of energy, accomplished by the production of glucose through actions on the liver. The added circulation of cortisol enhances the release of stored fat, turning fatty acids into available energy. Cortisol acts both directly and synergistically with *catecholamines* (stress hormones that are part of the SNS)—epinephrine and norepinephrine. Cortisol secretion potentiates the effect of these agents on degree and persistence of changes in vascular tone. Essentially, a response to stress has elements that are (a) immediate—through direct innervation of the cardiac myocytes; (b) intermediate—through releasing catecholamines into circulation; and (c) prolonged—through the enhancing effect of cortisol, both in duration and degree. In this way, the heart and vascular system can mount any range of response to the psychological stress that is perceived by the individual. Of course, because this type of stress is psychological, the perception of stress can persist in the absence of any real demand and thereby contribute to an unnecessarily prolonged and chronic response of the stress systems.

Epinephrine and norepinephrine also facilitate secondary effects of exposure to stressors beyond those on the heart, lungs, and large muscles. These effects include inhibition of stomach and upper-intestinal action to the point where digestion slows down or stops, blood vessels constrict in those parts of the body not involved in the response to the stressor, and blood vessels dilate in those muscles that are likely to be needed. In addition, because of receptors on blood platelets, there is an increase in platelet aggregability. Thus, in this coordinated response, the body is prepared for immediate action of a survival nature, sending blood to where it is needed and shunting it away from any unnecessary areas. In addition, the body prepares for injury, for example, by preparing the platelets to respond quickly in the event of a bleeding injury.

Psychological stress as such rarely requires a physical response. Indeed, many stressful circumstances—for example, those involving interpersonal stress such as work stress and relationship stress—require an inhibition of any physical response. Similarly, chronic life stress, such as that caused by poor living conditions, caregiver burden, and poor work conditions, has no "appropriate" response that can immediately terminate or reduce the degree of difficulty. Thus, under those conditions, the heart is prepared for action and the substances released into the circulation prepare for action, but the signal to the muscles is mixed. There is an increase in blood pressure due to an increase in CO but also due to an increase in systemic resistance—the blood vessels in the periphery in part constrict, and this pattern is mediated by elevated SNS activity and withdrawal of PNS influence. One consequence is an increase in turbulence within the coronary arteries, particularly at branch points, as the pressure within these vessels is increased. With that turbulence comes opportunities for acute injury to endothelial cells at the site of the turbulence, thereby setting the stage for the eventual development of a fatty streak and then onward to a plaque. In fact, research has shown that under controlled conditions, the performance of a stressful task such as serial subtraction or public speaking, or even the discussion of an event that previously provoked moderate to extreme anger, results in injury to, and death of, endothelial cells and a reduction in the ability of the body to restore these cells (Shimbo et al., 2013).

Poor recovery after exposure to acute psychological stress may be a marker of chronic autonomic imbalance—SNS hyperactivity and/or low vagal tone. This imbalance may persist and both potentiate and be sustained by continued stress, often in part due to cognitive rumination.

DISEASES OF THE HEART

It follows, after this description of the key components of the heart, that there are four major types of disease: coronary, valvular, electrical, and myopathic.

Coronary Atherosclerosis

Coronary atherosclerosis is an inflammatory disorder of the coronary arteries characterized by the development of both hard and soft plaques—

or *stenoses*—in the wall of the coronary arteries (see Figure 1.3). These plaques can grow to the point that they obstruct blood flow enough to cause *myocardial ischemia*, a condition characterized by insufficient blood flow to support the work of the heart; this often causes *angina pectoris*, the typical chest pain some patients with CHD experience during physical exertion. Even if not sufficiently obstructive to cause these symptoms, the plaque can be unstable or prone to rupture, and when this occurs, the subsequent outflow of plaque material into the coronary artery and consequent mounting of platelet aggregation causes a total obstruction of the vessel and an acute coronary syndrome (ACS) event.

Valvular Heart Disease

A second common type of cardiac disorder, *valvular heart disease*, is defined by the dysfunction of one or more cardiac valve and is characterized by the narrowing or obstruction of the valve opening (e.g., valvular stenosis or insufficiency) or leakage due to a failure of the valve leaflets to close properly (e.g., valvular regurgitation), resulting in the flow of blood back into the heart chamber from which it has just been ejected during chamber contraction. Valvular heart disease can be congenital, the result of infection such as rheumatic fever, or the result of the aging process.

Cardiac Arrhythmia

The third type of cardiac disorder, *cardiac arrhythmia*, is defined by dysfunction in the conduction system. This dysfunction can result in rapid (*tachycardia*) or slow (*bradycardia*) heart rate and/or a dyssynchrony in the sequence of one-to-one atrial and ventricular contractions. The danger in tachycardia is that it can lead to *fibrillation*, a rapid, irregular, and unsynchronized contraction of muscle fibers. When this occurs in the ventricle, it can lead to catastrophic arrhythmic death; even when it occurs in the atria (*atrial fibrillation*), it is not benign because it can cause pooling of blood in the atria, the formation of a clot, and then the freeing of that clot into the circulation, where it can cause a cerebrovascular event—a stroke.

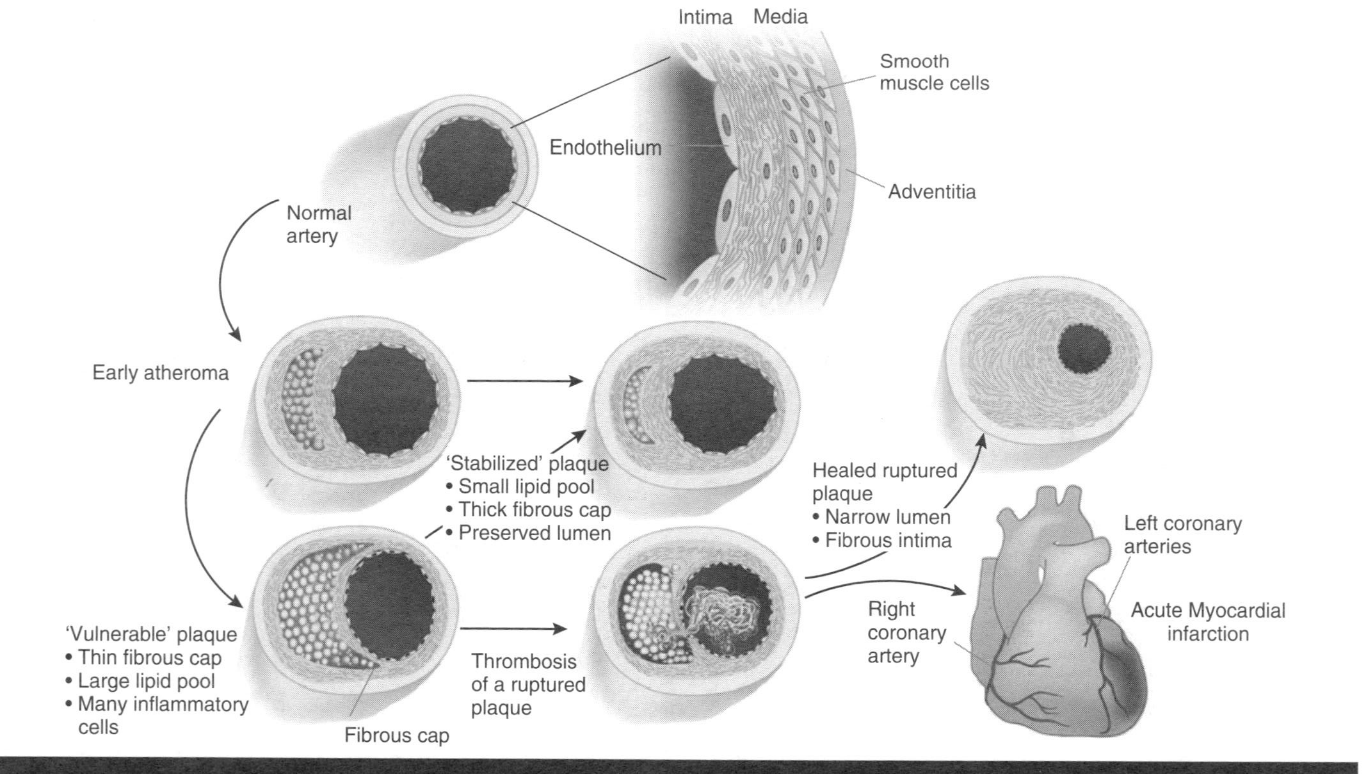

Figure 1.3

The process of coronary atherosclerosis and plaque development. Depiction of progressive coronary atherosclerosis—coronary artery disease. The cross-section of a healthy artery is seen at the top, depicting the layers of the artery, followed by progression of disease depicted by a progressively larger occlusion or plaque, which can become stable (i.e., with a thick fibrous cap) or vulnerable (i.e., with a thin cap and large lipid pool), ultimately leading to plaque rupture, thrombosis, and acute myocardial infarction. From "Inflammation in Atherosclerosis," by P. Libby, 2002, *Nature*, *420*, p. 872. Copyright 2002 by Macmillan Publishers: Nature. Reprinted with permission.

Cardiomyopathy and Heart Failure

The fourth type of cardiac disorder is defined by diseases of the heart muscle. In *cardiomyopathy*, the heart muscle becomes enlarged, thick, or rigid. As cardiomyopathy progresses, the heart becomes weaker and less able to pump blood effectively and efficiently. In addition, with this progressive dysfunction of the heart muscle, there is an accompanying failure to maintain a normal electrical rhythm, leading to cardiac arrhythmia. Cardiomyopathy also leads to heart failure (HF), which is in part characterized by a failure in heart pumping capacity; fluid buildup in the lungs, ankles, feet, legs, and/or abdomen; and problems with the heart valves. The most prevalent types of cardiomyopathy are hypertrophic, dilated, and restrictive.

Hypertrophic cardiomyopathy is common, can affect people of any age, and affects men and women equally. It happens when the heart muscle—usually the ventricles and septum—enlarge and thicken without any obvious cause. The thickened areas create narrowing in the ventricles, making it harder for the heart to pump blood. Hypertrophic cardiomyopathy also can cause stiffness of the ventricles, changes in the mitral valve, and cellular changes in the heart tissue.

Dilated cardiomyopathy develops when the ventricles enlarge and weaken. The condition usually starts in the left ventricle and, over time, can affect the right ventricle. The weakened chambers of the heart do not pump effectively, causing the heart muscle to work harder. Over time, the heart loses the ability to pump blood effectively, leading to HF, valvular disease, irregular heart rate, and blood clots in the heart chambers.

Restrictive cardiomyopathy develops when the ventricles become stiff and rigid but the walls of the heart do not thicken. As a result, the ventricles do not relax and do not fill normally. As the disease progresses, the ventricles do not pump as well, and the heart muscle weakens. Over time, restrictive cardiomyopathy also can lead to HF and valvular problems.

Some cardiomyopathy is unclassified and includes *takotsubo cardiomyopathy* (TCM), a condition also known as *broken heart syndrome.* This rare condition typically occurs in people after a major emotional shock, such as receiving unexpected news about the loss of a loved one.

It is, in part, characterized by failure of contraction in regional cardiac myocytes—*apical akinesis*—which results in the heart taking the shape of a Japanese gourd called a *takotsubo* for its use in capturing octopuses. It is also characterized by high circulating levels of catecholamines. Its rapid onset mimics ACS when the patient undergoes diagnostic cardiac angiography to determine the extent and severity of the expected blockages in the coronary arteries and left ventricular apical ballooning is found and there is no significant coronary artery stenosis. In most cases, this condition resolves in a matter of days—accompanied by a return of catecholamine levels to normal—with the heart assuming normal function. There have been cases of reported repeat TCM among a few individuals.

HF occurs when the heart (e.g., the left ventricle) is unable to pump blood forward into circulation with sufficient pressure and at a rate sufficient to meet the metabolic demands of the body. The clinical presentation can include fatigue, shortness of breath, and often *volume overload*—fluid buildup in the extremities and the lungs. It can be due to a "stiffening" of the left ventricle whereby the ventricle does not relax sufficiently after contraction and thus does not fill completely; the result is that there is not the full amount of blood to pump forward into circulation as would occur under normal circumstances, even though the percentage of blood pumped out of the ventricle when it contracts—the ejection fraction—remains within the normal range. This condition is called *heart failure with preserved ejection fraction*. HF can also be the final manifestation of the atherosclerotic process whereby the heart muscle is gradually weakened by recurrent ischemia and ACS events; here, the ejection fraction drops significantly—for example, from a normal 60% range to 35% or lower. Indeed, because ACS-related mortality has been greatly reduced by the emergence of effective medications and percutaneous interventions (see Chapter 4), there has been a gradual increase in the incidence of HF and its related, acute manifestation of congestive heart failure.

Having provided this overview of the cardiovascular system and diseases of the heart, we now move to a presentation of etiology and sociocultural factors related to heart disease.

2

Etiology and Sociocultural Factors Related to Heart Disease

Atherosclerosis, a primary cause of coronary heart disease (CHD), is a progressive process that starts with an insult to the interior lining of an artery—to the endothelial cells—and ends with blockages sufficient to impair blood flow. Endothelial cells in healthy arteries perform a range of metabolic and signaling functions that maintain vessel homeostasis. Endothelial cells also modulate an immune response and thereby resist local inflammation. However, when these cells are injured locally, a process is engaged whereby inflammatory cytokines are activated and a cascade of events ensue that can lead to the development of fatty streaks, the engagement and migration of smooth muscle cells from the media to the intima, and onward to the development of atherosclerotic plaques.

A *fatty streak* is the original lesion of atherosclerosis and can be found in the aorta and coronary arteries of most people over the age of 20. It does not protrude into the artery lumen and, although the cause remains

http://dx.doi.org/10.1037/0000070-003
Psychological Treatment of Cardiac Patients, by M. M. Burg

to be fully determined, various stimuli, including cigarette smoking, a high-fat diet, elevated lipid levels, and psychological stress, cause endothelial dysfunction, and such dysfunction allows entry and modification of lipids into the subendothelial space. This provokes an inflammatory response that first shows up as the fatty streak. At the cellular level, the barrier properties of the endothelium are disrupted, inflammatory cytokines are released, leukocytes are recruited from the circulation, normal antithrombotic processes are disrupted, and the ongoing release of vasodilatory nitric oxide is altered. Thus, injury to the endothelium and the resulting endothelial dysfunction represent the initiating events of atherosclerosis.

With the failure of barrier properties, low-density lipoprotein (LDL) cholesterol particles enter the intimal space, where they undergo oxidation. In addition, recruitment of leukocytes leads to the attraction of a type of white blood cell called a *monocyte*, which expresses high levels of inflammatory cytokines such as interleukin-1 and tumor necrosis factor alpha. After monocytes penetrate the intima, they are transformed into macrophages that incorporate the now resident LDL particles and become foam cells that further accumulate in the now growing plaque. Although *apoptosis* (cell death) of these foam cells is a normal and associated process, there is a failure to sufficiently clear these dead foam cells, thereby promoting the accumulation of cellular debris, which forms the lipid-rich, necrotic core of the plaque. During years of development, the atherosclerotic plaque grows, becoming defined by a thrombogenic lipid core surrounded by a protective fibrous and calcified cap. The integrity of the fibrous cap is a function of the balance between development by smooth muscle cells and breakdown by enzymes.

Early plaque growth involves a compensatory process whereby there is an outward "remodeling" of the vessel wall that serves to maintain the diameter of the lumen. Although these lesions thus do not affect blood flow (e.g., in the coronary arteries) and do not cause symptoms, they may be "hot" and unstable (e.g., highly inflammatory and with only a thin fibrous cap). Because they do not protrude into the lumen or obstruct blood flow, they are asymptomatic and escape detection; even if they were symptomatic, they would escape detection during coronary angiography because they do not reduce the lumen in size. Nonetheless, these hot and unstable plaques can rupture and cause an instantaneous formation of a thrombus (blood clot) that fully occludes the vessel lumen and results in an acute coronary syndrome (ACS) event.

Over decades, the lipid core grows, eventually causing the plaque to protrude into the arterial lumen. There the cap is exposed to mechanical stresses at the plaque border, in part due to the flow of blood around the lesion and in part due to coronary artery *vasomotion*, or transition through states of relative dilation and constriction. The thickness of the cap and the degree of inflammation and content of the necrotic core define the vulnerability of the plaque to rupture under a range of conditions that include even moderate anger and psychological stress, cocaine and marijuana use, and catastrophic events such as natural disasters and war.

ISCHEMIC HEART DISEASE

Although the long-standing focus in clinical cardiology has been on the symptoms produced by a large, flow-limiting obstruction in the coronary artery, approximately one half of patients with coronary atherosclerosis have no symptoms of the disease, and this can include patients with coronary artery stenosis of 90% occlusion or greater, as long as compensatory collaterals maintain sufficient blood flow to support the contraction of the cardiac myocytes regardless of the demand placed on the heart. Indeed, it is for this reason so many ACS events are unexpected—because there were no prior symptoms. Once symptoms are present, however, the condition comes to be called *ischemic heart disease* (IHD), a condition in which there is an imbalance between myocardial oxygen supply, provided by the blood circulating through the coronary arteries and downwind coronary microvascular bed, and demand for oxygen that results from contractile work being done. In the normal heart, the oxygen requirements of the heart are continually matched by the coronary arterial supply system. Even during vigorous physical activity when oxygen demands are highest, the balance is maintained by the compensatory mechanisms that increase blood flow through the capillaries. This ability to increase flow is essential because, unlike most tissues, the heart extracts almost all the oxygen from blood even at the basal state. Thus, the additional oxygen requirement caused by exertion can only be met by an autoregulatory process that increases blood flow.

The reduction in blood flow that accompanies coronary atherosclerosis is largely a function of the reduction in vessel diameter caused by obstruction of the coronary lumen by a plaque. When the plaque reduces the diameter by greater than 70%, there is a sharp reduction in maximal possible blood flow, regardless of the degree to which the arterioles and coronary microcirculation try to compensate—only so much blood can pass through the blocked arterial segment. Thus, when demand exceeds the ability to increase supply, myocardial ischemia ensues. It is important to note, however, that the degree of stenosis is not the only factor involved in the occurrence of ischemia. Endothelial dysfunction, particularly at the site of a fatty streak or nonobstructive lesion, can cause inappropriate vasoconstriction, thereby further reducing the lumen diameter; this has in particular been observed during psychological stress. In addition, in a phenomenon called *coronary microvascular disease*, there is a failure of autoregulatory processes so that the capillary bed does not allow the required increase in blood flow. These two processes underscore an emerging understanding that IHD is not necessarily the same thing as obstructive coronary disease.

There is a spectrum of clinical presentations that accompany IHD, including stable angina, unstable angina, silent ischemia, coronary microvascular disease (often called syndrome X), and ACS.

Chronic stable angina presents as a predictable pattern of transient chest discomfort that occurs during physical exertion or emotional stress. Different patients experience a choking sensation in the upper chest and throat, pain in the jaw, burning in the ears, shoulder, arm, or back discomfort, and exertional indigestion or belching. The range of symptoms is believed to be due to the joining in the spine of nerves innervating the heart, arms, thorax, abdomen, and head and the resulting difficulty of the brain to distinguish the source of the pain signals. This explains why some patients having an ACS event think they have indigestion.

Chronic stable angina is caused by fixed plaques in one or more coronary arteries, with the pattern of symptoms correlated with the degree of overall stenotic burden. With the increase in heart rate, blood pressure, and ventricular contractile force—mediated by the sympathetic nervous system—that accompanies exertion or stress, there is an increase in the consumption of oxygen by the heart muscle and thus an increase in oxygen demand. The presence of obstructive stenoses interferes with the ability to increase blood flow and oxygen supply. The myocytes are starved of oxygen, resulting in a change in metabolic characteristics from aerobic to anaerobic, the accumulation of metabolic by-products, and ultimately a failure of contraction within groups of myocytes—called the *ischemic cascade*. Each step of this process is amenable to a particular diagnostic technique described later. However, at the symptom level, this cascade culminates with the experience of characteristic angina symptoms. Also, as noted earlier, the reduction in blood flow that accompanies a fixed plaque-related obstruction can be augmented due to transient endothelial or coronary microvascular dysfunction. What characterizes chronic stable angina is the predictable pattern (e.g., a given patient will predictably experience angina symptoms under a given level of physical exertion or psychologically stressful circumstances).

Unstable angina pectoris (UAP) is defined by a sudden increase in the occurrence and duration of angina events in a patient who to that point had a predictable pattern of these experiences. Angina is now occurring at a lower level of physical exertion or psychological stress or perhaps even at rest. This now unstable angina can be a precursor to myocardial infarction (MI) and, indeed, together MI and UAP are subsumed under the designation of ACS events, which result most commonly from rupture of an unstable atherosclerotic plaque with subsequent platelet aggregation and thrombosis.

Silent ischemia describes a transient imbalance between myocardial oxygen supply and demand that occurs in the absence of angina symptoms.

It has been observed to account for up to 75% of discrete ischemic events in patients with chronic stable angina, but can also occur in patients without any anginal symptoms. In this absence of an anginal warning system (e.g., no symptoms to warn patients so they can address the symptoms with their physician or, if already diagnosed, take appropriate medications), the patient is at elevated risk of an ACS event. It should be noted that silent ischemia is not necessarily a function of overall stenotic burden or the degree of blockage in a given coronary artery; it can occur regardless of these anatomical features. In addition, when ischemia has been provoked by psychological stress under controlled laboratory conditions—so-called *mental stress ischemia* (MSI)—it is almost universally silent.

Coronary microvascular disease and *syndrome X* are terms used to describe anginal symptoms in patients who do not have obstructive coronary atherosclerosis but who might demonstrate evidence of ischemia, such as changes in the electrocardiogram (ECG) or impairment in left ventricular function on standard diagnostic tests. This condition is often due to inadequate vasodilator reserve of the coronary capillary bed—a failure of the arterioles to dilate and thus increase blood flow to the capillaries, hence the descriptive name. Although this condition predominates among women, it is not altogether uncommon among men. Furthermore, evidence has suggested that this condition may in part underlie the occurrence of MSI.

Acute coronary syndrome events are a class of life-threatening conditions that form a continuum from UAP to acute MI. More than 90% of ACS events are the consequence of plaque rupture with subsequent platelet aggregation and thrombus formation. With the formation of thrombus, what had been an area of lumen narrowing due to a stenosis becomes a near-total or total occlusion. A partially occlusive thrombus then causes either UAP or non-ST-elevation MI (NSTEMI), with the latter distinguished by consequent myocardial necrosis—death of cardiac muscle tissue due to oxygen starvation. A fully occlusive thrombus results in the more severe ST-elevation-MI (STEMI) and a larger area of cardiac necrosis. The time from initial near total or total occlusion to irreversible and proliferated effects occurs in minutes; thus, the sooner a patient can get to the cardiac catheterization lab for an intervention to open the now occluded vessel, the more myocardium can be salvaged. Hence the metric "door to balloon time"—the time from arriving at the emergency department of a hospital to being in the cardiac catheterization lab with an intervention underway—and the rubric "time is myocardium."

With necrosis of regional heart muscle—the area that had been served by the coronary artery distribution distal or "downwind" of the MI site—is a process of remodeling and the development of scar. The greater the area of cell death and scar, the greater the compromise in ventricular function because now the ventricular wall does not contract as fully and uniformly as it had before the ACS event. A drop in the left ventricular ejection fraction ensues, and this can eventually lead to valvular issues, heart failure, and cardiac arrhythmia.

In addition to the characteristic symptoms of ischemia that accompany ACS, there are key diagnostic features. These include abnormalities in the ECG waveform (e.g., ST-segment depression and/or T-wave inversion with UAP or NSTEMI; ST-segment elevation evolving into T-wave inversion with STEMI) and the presence of cardiac-specific markers of cellular necrosis in the circulating blood (e.g., troponin I and T). Imaging modalities such as cardiac ultrasound (echocardiography) are also occasionally used to identify new ventricular dysfunction when the ECG and serum markers are uncertain.

ACS-related complications can include death and further progression of the infarction. These and other complications can result from the inflammatory, mechanical, and electrical or conduction abnormalities that are a consequence of regional cardiac necrosis. There can be recurrent ischemia; potentially fatal (ventricular) and nonfatal cardiac arrhythmias (e.g., because the location of necrosis involves the passage of key components of the conduction system or because of the amount of myocardium involved in the ACS); heart failure or cardiogenic shock, a condition of severely decreased cardiac contraction and hence output (i.e., very low systolic blood pressure) that often occurs when the area of infarct involves 40% or greater of the left ventricular mass; and papillary muscle rupture, another potentially fatal accompaniment of ACS.

IMPACT OF HEART DISEASE ON VULNERABLE OR DISPARATE GROUPS

Age-adjusted cardiac mortality for African Americans in the United States is 33% higher than for the population as a whole (Mensah & Brown, 2007). Hispanics/Latinos have a lower risk of cardiac mortality and lower prevalence of CHD compared with non-Hispanics, but the finding is paradoxical in that the population also shows a worse cardiovascular risk profile (Balfour, Ruiz, Talavera, Allison, & Rodriguez, 2016). It is difficult to make generalizations about the Hispanic/Latino subgroup because the population is diverse, including Puerto Ricans, Dominicans, Cubans, and Mexicans as well as South and Central Americans. There are also substantial differences between racial and ethnic subgroups regarding the onset and trajectory of disease. For example, African Americans are more likely to have an earlier onset of disease and are more likely to die from heart disease. They are less likely to receive appropriate and/or timely treatments for heart disease—or risk factors—in the United States. Even when variation in risk factor differences, appropriateness of the cardiac procedure, socioeconomic status, and/or insurance are controlled for in analyses, they are less likely to be diagnosed or to be offered aspirin, a prime pharmacologic agent for prevention and treatment, prophylactically or after a cardiac event, and they wait longer for angioplasty (Davis, Vinci, Okwuosa, Chase, & Huang, 2007).

Low socioeconomic status (SES) is overrepresented in racial and ethnic subgroups, making it difficult to disentangle the relative contribution of poverty to racial disparities in cardiac health (Adler et al., 1994). Lower SES is associated with an overall more stressful and less healthy environment, higher likelihood of exposure to traumatic incidents, difficulty accessing high-quality sources of nutrition, reduced access to physical fitness facilities and safe exercise environments (e.g., safe streets for walking), and barriers to accessing specialty health care (Phillips & Klein, 2010). Low SES is correlated with delays in treatment seeking, illiteracy, and critical knowledge gaps (e.g., how to take medication; Kaplan, Spittel, & David, 2015).

The paucity of adequate data is one of the greatest barriers to understanding why disparities in cardiovascular morbidity and mortality exist. Without such data, it is difficult to fully understand how the etiology of heart disease differs between underserved subgroups or to develop a plan to address cardiovascular health disparities. Targeted research will play a key role in improving the rates and outcomes of CHD in minority populations.

CARDIOVASCULAR BEHAVIORAL MEDICINE: A HISTORY OF BEHAVIORAL CARDIOLOGY RESEARCH

Although the past several decades have been accompanied by rapid progress in the medical treatment of heart disease, most notably in the development of new drugs and advances in approaches to coronary revascularization, that has in many ways eclipsed the focus on the psychological and psychosocial domains, the importance of psychosocial factors to CHD—the mind–body connection—has been appreciated since the time of the great Greek physician Celsus (1935/1971), to whom the quote "Fear and anger and any other state of mind may often be apt to excite the pulse" has been attributed. In the 18th century, John Hunter, a Scottish surgeon and one of the most distinguished scientists and surgeons of his day, was noted to have said, "My life is in the hands of any rascal who chooses to put me in a passion," (as cited in DeBakey & Gotto, 1977) because of the chest pain he would experience under such circumstances, likely—as he understood—due to underlying CHD. He died suddenly in 1793 after participating in a violent argument at a faculty meeting, and in a series of lectures at the turn of the 20th century, Sir William Osler described the circumstances of Hunter's death, noting, "In silent rage and in the next room he gave a deep groan and fell down dead" (as cited in DeBakey & Gotto, 1977). In these lectures, Osler (1910) went on to state, "It is not the delicate person who is prone to angina, but the robust, the vigorous in mind and body, the keen and ambitious man, the indicator of whose engines is always at 'full speed ahead'" (p. 839).

The literature contains many such anecdotal reports that both implicitly and explicitly describe a contribution of psychological factors to CHD, yet it was only during the mid-20th century that programs of research were developed to characterize this contribution and to do so in a way that was actionable. In particular, it was two cardiologists in San Francisco,

Ray Rosenman and Meyer Friedman, who noted certain characteristics of their patients. These characteristics appeared to be defined by what they came to call *hurry sickness*—an insatiable time pressure to do more and more, coupled with an experience of the world as consisting of obstacles to one's efforts (Friedman & Rosenman, 1974). These obstacles required a high degree of continuous vigilance so as to identify and overcome them quickly, and because these obstacles interfered with a need or drive to accomplishment, the response to them was hostile and aggressive. Rosenman and Friedman came to call this constellation of factors "behavior pattern A," which later evolved into Type A behavior pattern, and unfortunately, Type A personality. What made this evolution unfortunate was that the focus on observable behavior was lost. Indeed, being good clinicians, Rosenman and Friedman developed a structured clinical interview and defined the relative presence of Type A behavior pattern by the responses by patients to a set of questions, not just in the content of their responses but also in the manner of their response, using voice, facial expression, choice of words, and strong hand gestures to define the relative presence of the behavior pattern.

In a program of research that spanned from the mid-1950s to the mid-1980s, the research of these cardiologists and others demonstrated that the Type A behavior pattern was independently associated with incident CHD and CHD-related mortality and with behavioral risk factors that contributed to CHD (e.g., tobacco and alcohol use). They further demonstrated that a group-delivered and stress management–based intervention could reduce this behavior pattern and the rate of recurrent cardiac events. Related efforts were directed toward the identification of the key elements of the Type A behavior constellation that contributed to CHD risk, and this work identified hostility and anger as particularly toxic. Work during the 1990s by researchers at Harvard University hospitals revealed that the experience of a single episode of moderate to extreme anger could trigger an ACS event, with the risk being present for up to 2 hours after the experience of anger and being additive; that is, if another such incident occurred during the 2-hour hazard period, the risk was compounded. Others found that the relating of an event that provoked such anger could cause a transient narrowing of the coronary arteries at the site of even minor blockages (Yeung et al., 1991) and that with this narrowing there was a significant reduction in blood reaching the heart muscle (Krantz & Burg, 2014). Of note, in almost all cases, this impairment in blood flow was not accompanied by symptoms of angina—the characteristic chest pain—thus robbing patients of the warning signs they could self-treat with appropriate medications (e.g., nitroglycerin tablet).

Research on Type A behavior, hostility, and anger was slowly abandoned as efforts to replicate failed. This failure has been attributed in part to a "drift" in the underlying conceptualization and the movement away from the more difficult clinical interview to the self-administered questionnaire. In essence, something else was being measured. Efforts to prevent and treat CHD were also changing—for example, with the implementation of aspirin therapy and the use of statin medications to treat high cholesterol. These treatments may have altered the physiological pathway(s) by which psychological factors contribute to CHD incidence and recurrence—for example, by reducing the aggregation of platelets when a plaque in the coronary artery ruptures or by reducing the inflammatory state that underlies coronary blockages. In support of this hypothesis, the researchers who demonstrated that anger could trigger an ACS event also found that if the patient was taking aspirin, the risk of this occurring was largely eliminated.

As research on Type A behavior and CHD was dissipating, a new focus on depression arose. From the late 1980s to the present, depression, as both a diagnostic entity and a subsyndromal index of symptom severity, has become a significant target of research on psychological factors and CHD. Although some questions remain, the great majority of the research continues to show that a lifetime history of depression increases the risk of incident CHD and that, among patients who have experienced an ACS event, even a relatively low threshold of depression symptom severity increases the risk of early recurrence and mortality (Carney & Freedland, 2008; Frasure-Smith & Lesperance, 2005; van Melle et al., 2004). As with Type A, depression can be thought of as a constellation of characteristics entailing affective symptoms, somatic symptoms, and cognitive symptoms. Some argue that depression reflects CHD severity—that it is the somatic symptoms that carry CHD-related risk and that these symptoms reflect the severity of cardiac dysfunction. Researchers typically control for CHD severity statistically, yet depression still predicts outcome, carrying up to 2.5-fold increased risk of ACS recurrence and mortality (van Melle et al., 2004). As research has progressed, population subsets have been discerned—that is, incident depression that occurs at the time of the ACS event as a first episode of depression at a relatively late life stage versus the more traditional remitting recurrent depression with the first incident at early adulthood. In addition, the pathways by which depression increases ACS recurrence and mortality risk have been an important research focus, identifying (medication) adherence, anhedonia, and inflammation as potentially important.

The *randomized clinical trial* (RCT)—a clinical trial in which participants are randomly assigned to separate groups that compare different treatments—is the gold standard for assessing whether a particular treatment is beneficial for a defined outcome. Although a great deal of research has shown that psychosocial factors increase the risk of early incident CHD and ACS events and contribute to event recurrence and mortality, the breadth and depth of this literature are not matched by a body of clinical trials literature. In addition to the depression RCTs and the Rosenman and Friedman Type A behavior RCTs, there have been trials that focused more generally on stress reduction, and these have shown promise. For example, a stress management intervention that included relaxation training, cognitive reframing of stress-inducing thoughts and evaluations of ongoing circumstances surrounding the patient, and skills training to reduce the affective and behavioral aspects of stress experience and responding was successful in reducing the occurrence of ischemia in the natural environment and during stress testing among patients with heart disease (Blumenthal et al., 2002). This approach has also met with success in other trials that have also shown a reduction in long-term mortality (Orth-Gomér et al., 2009). More research is needed to provide a sufficient evidence base that can guide the care of the cardiac patient in the modern age, where standard medical therapy has already significantly reduced incidence and recurrence rate.

With these reviews completed, we now move from a discussion of what can go wrong to a presentation of the various treatment approaches that have been developed to address CHD.

3

Medical Treatment of Heart Disease

Medical treatment of heart disease can be remarkably complex, involving multiple concurrent medications designed to bolster cardiac function while alleviating stress on the heart, along with medications that directly address constituent risk factors such as elevated blood pressure, cholesterol, and blood sugar. Treatment can also include a host of diagnostic and interventional methods to, on the one hand, pinpoint the issues with the heart and cardiovascular system and, on the other hand, directly affect the associated disease process(es). Once again, it is essential for the psychologist to have a full and conversant understanding of these treatments to be able to interact as a peer with other health care providers, while understanding and appreciating the experience of the patient and family.

A patient's medical history, a physical examination, and both routine and specialized cardiovascular diagnostic tests are used to identify the

http://dx.doi.org/10.1037/0000070-004
Psychological Treatment of Cardiac Patients, by M. M. Burg

presence of coronary heart disease (CHD) and determine the best treatment. The medical history includes the patient's chief complaint, how long symptoms have been present, and activities that exacerbate or improve the symptoms (e.g., physical activity, eating, reclining, stress). In patients with symptoms of angina pectoris, the quality of the symptom (sharp, dull, constricting, burning) and the quantity of time it is experienced (minutes, hours, days) are particularly important. Routine laboratory tests include a chest X-ray to determine heart size (enlarged in cardiomyopathy) and the presence of fluid (associated with heart failure) and blood work to identify possible infections, electrolyte disturbances, and blood sugar and lipid levels. More specialized blood work may involve measurement of inflammation, particularly high sensitivity C-reactive protein. Combining these findings with a review of risk-related behaviors (e.g., sedentary lifestyle, tobacco use) and associated features (e.g., blood pressure, age, gender) allows for the application of risk stratification models (e.g., Framingham Risk Score; Wannamethee, Shaper, Lennon, & Morris, 2005) that help guide risk-reduction efforts and pharmacologic treatment (e.g., for hypertension, diabetes, high cholesterol). The risk score can also guide the advisability of further and more specific diagnostic testing. Specialized cardiovascular diagnostic tests include resting and ambulatory electrocardiogram (ECG), stress test with either nuclear or ultrasound imaging, computed tomography (CT) angiography, cardiac MRI, and coronary catheterization.

The *ECG* (also called *EKG*) is a quick and inexpensive test that provides an enormous amount of information. A 12-lead arrangement with leads fastened at various points along the chest provides electrical vectors representing different physical locations in and around the surface of the heart. The resulting waveforms represent aspects of the cardiac cycle that repeat with each heartbeat and that are designated by letters *P*, *Q*, *R*, *S*, and *T*; specific patterns observed between these distinct wave points indicate the heart rate and rhythm, the presence of ischemia, heart chamber enlargement, thickening of the muscle walls, and the presence and location of muscle damage due to prior acute coronary syndrome (ACS) events.

The ECG can also be performed over an extended period in the natural environment (e.g., for 24 hours) through the use of a *Holter monitor*.

This digital recording device to which the ECG leads are connected allows for the assessment of the heart rhythm and waveform as the patient goes about routine activity. The Holter monitor is most often used for the assessment of rhythm disturbances such as atrial fibrillation. In research, the combination of the Holter monitor with an electronic diary has been used to determine both the daily frequency of myocardial ischemia and the precipitating events (e.g., emotional stress or physical exertion occurring proximally before an ischemic ECG change).

Stress tests typically involve a patient walking on a treadmill or pedaling on a stationary bicycle, in each case with increasing effort (e.g., speeding up the treadmill and increasing the incline, according to a rigorous time-based protocol), and during this physical exertion, the ECG is continuously monitored. The endpoints of a maximal stress test are development of anginal symptoms, an abnormal change in blood pressure, changes on the ECG, or reaching 85% of the maximum predicted heart rate (220 minus the patient's age). As long as the patient is exercised sufficiently so that the peak heart rate during the stress test is at least 85% of what is predicted for age, the stress test is reasonably accurate in diagnosing significant CHD and a near-term prognosis. Markedly abnormal ECG changes at an early stage of exercise, prolonged ST-segment changes after stopping exercise, major cardiac arrhythmias during exercise, and having to stop the test early are all markers of higher risk of myocardial infarction (MI). Given its ease and low cost, this arrangement is excellent for screening and can frequently be repeated to assess the effect of interventions such as exercise training and medications for angina, arrhythmia, or elevated blood pressure. Although the use of the ECG for stress testing is inexpensive and noninvasive and does not involve injections or radiation exposure, it has up to a 25% false negative and positive rate, with even worse performance among women (Fletcher et al., 2017). Moreover, a patient must physically be able to exercise.

Nuclear stress tests (e.g., with the radioisotopes technetium or sestamibi) were devised to improve the accuracy of CHD diagnosis. Instead of assessing ECG changes with exercise, these studies evaluate distribution of a radioactive tracer isotope (*myocardial perfusion imaging* [MPI]) that is "tagged" to red blood cells perfusing the heart through the coronary arteries. Images of myocardial perfusion are obtained at rest and following stress (e.g., exercise or administration of a vasoactive drug). With computer software, color images representing perfusion in multiple "slices" of the heart in three dimensions along the long and short axes are created, and the rest and stress images are compared to assess decreased perfusion with stress. Reduction of blood flow—flow defects—can be localized by the area of decreased perfusion, and on the basis of standard anatomy, the location of these flow defects can be attributed to problems—stenosis—in specific coronary artery distributions. Software also creates a dynamic image of the left ventricle beating, thus showing poorly or noncontracting segments and generating a quantitative left ventricular ejection fraction (LVEF). This form of stress testing provides substantially greater accuracy than the ECG, with only 10% false negatives and positives, and can identify the presence and extent of scars from a prior MI and the location and severity of ischemia. They thus can identify the highest risk patients who need immediate and aggressive medical and/or interventional therapy (angioplasty or stent or bypass surgery). The disadvantages are that they are more expensive, expose the patient to radiation (limiting frequent studies), and take several hours to complete.

Positron emission tomography (PET) is another useful nuclear test that can measure not only myocardial perfusion but also metabolic activity. It can thereby be useful to determine whether a given area of the left ventricle is still viable (i.e., still metabolically active) after ACS events when other tests show no movement during the heartbeat in that particular area. This information is useful for determining whether to perform a revascularization procedure (angioplasty or bypass surgery) to restore blood flow to the affected region. PET is also used to assess function of the coronary microvascular bed in suspected microvascular disease, using a measurement called *coronary flow reserve.*

Cardiac ultrasound (or echocardiogram [ECHO]) is a noninvasive technique that uses sound waves to assess global heart function during relaxation (diastole) and contraction (systole). There are two approaches to the use of ECHO: *transthoracic* (TTE), in which the ECHO probe is variably placed on the chest at different locations so as to sonographically visualize the heart from different angles, and *transesophageal* (TEE), in which the probe is placed down the esophagus. The advantage of TEE over TTE is that it provides clearer images, especially of structures that are difficult to view through the chest wall. This is because the heart rests directly on the esophagus, leaving only millimeters that the ultrasound beam has to travel. ECHO is useful for identifying wall motion abnormalities (areas of reduced movement or nor movement), myocardial hypertrophy (thickening), valvular dysfunction, and presence of clots, tumors, or other anatomical irregularities.

ECHO can also be used in the setting of a stress test, thereby providing the same assessments of the heart under conditions of demand. When used in this way, a set of resting images is first obtained. The patient is then exercised on treadmill or bike (or a pharmacologic agent is used to induce demand conditions). At peak stress, the patient is taken from the treadmill or bike, and another set of images is obtained, thereby assessing whether stress compromises heart function. ECHO stress tests have a lower predictive accuracy than nuclear perfusion imaging for detecting myocardial ischemia; however, there is no radiation exposure, and the test takes a shorter time to perform.

CT angiography uses a combination of electron beams (X-rays) and computer analysis of the resulting data to provide detailed images of the coronary arteries and can thus be used to identify blockages with some precision. Furthermore, because of the radiopaque nature of calcium, a major constituent of bone, the calcium content of these blockages can be measured with some precision. From this is derived an overall calcium score, a measure that has been found to be predictive of incident ACS events, likely because the score represents the degree of stenoses throughout the coronary artery "tree," and the more stenoses, the greater the risk that any one stenosis will rupture and cause an ACS event. Although this overall noninvasive and relatively inexpensive test offers an important new element to the diagnosis of CHD, it has not replaced the use of coronary angiography, which has greater precision.

Cardiac MRI has applications for visualizing aspects of cardiac anatomy such as cardiac chambers and wall thickness. Furthermore, when used in concert with an injectable contrast agent, it is a superior method for assessing myocardial viability, compared with, for example, PET. Assessment of post-ACS left ventricular scarring visualized using a method called *delayed-contrast MRI* can provide important data for prediction of sudden cardiac death.

Overall, the clinical use of these imaging methods has greatly reduced the need for invasive cardiac catheterization to identify plaque volume and location, thus identifying the high-risk patient in need of angioplasty or bypass surgery and/or aggressive pharmacologic therapy and lifestyle intervention.

Cardiac catheterization is the gold standard for assessing coronary atherosclerosis. It involves the threading of a small-gauge plastic catheter via the arteries and veins of the legs or arms, through the aorta, and into the ostia (the takeoff point) of the right and left coronary arteries. A radiopaque dye is injected, and moving picture X-ray images are obtained as the contrast moves through the right and left coronary artery "trees" with each heartbeat (i.e., from the left main coronary artery and down through the left anterior descending coronary artery with associated diagonals, and left circumflex coronary artery with associated marginal), thus revealing blockages that are visualized as changes in the diameter of the imaged vessel. By repeat injections and capturing images at different angles, the coronary arteries can be visualized in three dimensions. When combined with information from MPI, for example, the presence of a large blockage in a coronary arterial distribution that has a perfusion defect with stress—a so-called culprit lesion—can be immediately addressed through the use of angioplasty, with or without stent (discussed later). Additional information about whether a given stenosis is flow limiting or highly inflammatory and thus at higher risk of rupture can be obtained through the use of specialized intravascular ultrasound or fractional flow reserve probes. In addition, pressure-sensitive probes can be used to determine the severity of aortic stenosis, whereas the injection of contrast directly into the left ventricle provides for assessment of LVEF. Once diagnosed, CHD can be treated through behavioral risk factor modification or pharmacotherapy and/or interventionally through angioplasty (percutaneous coronary intervention) or surgery (coronary artery bypass graft).

HEALTH RISK BEHAVIOR CHANGE

Because a great degree of chronic disease burden can be attributed to lifestyle and stress, health risk behavior change is key in treating CHD. The contribution of health risk behavior and related psychological factors to chronic CHD burden has been estimated at 40%, according to a 2010 Institute of Medicine Report (Fuster & Kelly, 2010). Health risk behavior includes poor diet, tobacco use, physical inactivity, and excess alcohol use. In addition, the INTERHEART study (Rosengren et al., 2004; Yusuf et al., 2004), a case-control analysis of factors associated with risk of acute MI across 52 countries and including over 24,000 patients, found that abnormal lipids, smoking, hypertension, diabetes, abdominal obesity, psychosocial factors, consumption of alcohol, and lack of regular physical activity and inadequate consumption of fruits and vegetables account for most of the risk of myocardial infarction worldwide in both sexes and at all ages in all regions. Furthermore, the presence of psychosocial stressors, defined as depression, perceived stress at home or work, low locus of control, and major life events, was associated with increased risk of MI. Interpreting these data, the authors concluded that approaches aimed at modifying these factors should be developed.

Whether a patient has chronic stable CHD, has recently experienced an ACS event or revascularization, has recently gotten an implantable cardioverter defibrillator, or presents with any other cardiac condition, a first step is a thorough assessment of overall risk factor status, with a particular focus on behavioral and psychosocial risk factors. In particular, cessation of smoking is perhaps the most important aspect of health risk reduction. Similarly, chronic alcohol or substance abuse should be identified and addressed. An assessment of depression, anxiety, and general chronic and acute stress should be made, and this can be done using a number of available questionnaire and interview protocols that are discussed later. A thorough case conceptualization that considers multiple health risk behaviors and their interaction should lead to a discussion with the patient focused on treatment priorities, followed by the implementation of an overall strategy that relies on the pragmatic and behavior-focused approaches shown to be most effective with medical populations. For some patients, treatment with psychoactive medications may be indicated, and the use of these agents as indicated should be managed by physicians who are trained in their use with cardiac patients. A more complete discussion of these approaches is found in later sections.

Pharmacotherapy

Treatment for patients with CHD often includes the chronic use of a range of medications. These include antiplatelet agents (e.g., aspirin), agents to reduce the demand on the heart (e.g., beta-blockers), agents to relax the blood vessels (e.g., calcium channel blockers [CCBs], angiotensin converting enzyme [ACE] inhibitors), agents that acutely dilate blood vessels (e.g., nitroglycerin), and lipid-lowering agents (e.g., statins). Low-dose (81 mg) aspirin is also used for primary prevention—for example, among individuals with a positive family history of CHD and multiple risk factors. In patients with documented CHD or after ACS a higher dose is often used (e.g., 325 mg). Beta-blockers work by blocking sympathetic nervous system (SNS) receptors, thus attenuating the associated input; this works to attenuate the increase in heart rate and contractility brought on by physical exertion and psychological stress. Beta-blockers are also a first-line therapy for treating heart failure. CCBs also work through SNS-related pathways, whereas ACE inhibitors work through the renin–angiotensin–aldosterone pathway. These agents are also used for the treatment of hypertension because of their effects on blood pressure.

Percutaneous Coronary Intervention

Revascularization—treatments to restore flow to blocked coronary arteries—can be accomplished through both percutaneous and surgical means.

Percutaneous coronary interventions (PCIs) are the most commonly performed medical procedures in the United States and are performed by interventional cardiologists (those who perform coronary angiography) using a percutaneous cardiac catheterization technique. As described earlier, a catheter is threaded to the affected coronary artery from the groin, arm, or wrist. A wire is passed beyond the site of blockage, and a balloon along this wire is first situated adjacent to the blockage and then inflated, compressing the plaque and thereby substantially reducing the degree of blockage. Patients may experience chest discomfort when the balloon is inflated. A scaffold-like structure—a *stent*—is also often used to help maintain the opening the balloon created.

With a growing understanding of the biology underlying plaque proliferation, drug-eluting stents have been developed. These slowly release pharmacologic agents to block cell proliferation and prevent fibrosis that could otherwise over time block the stented artery (*restenosis*). When drug-eluting stents are used in a PCI, a patient is placed on an antiplatelet agent (e.g., Plavix) to address the increased risk of thrombus formation and ACS that accompanies the use of these stents. When balloon angioplasty is used alone, plaque restenosis occurs in up to 30% of cases. When a bare metal stent or a drug-eluting stent is used, the restenosis rate is reduced to 10%. Thus, PCI with stenting is the procedure of choice in larger vessels, whereas in smaller vessels PCI without stenting is preferred because small stents are not available. PCI has a serious complication rate of less than 1% for vascular injury, with serious bleeding occurring in fewer than 5% of patients. It typically involves an overnight hospital stay postprocedure.

Coronary Artery Bypass Graft Surgery

Surgical revascularization—*coronary artery bypass grafting* (CABG)—is an invasive procedure. The procedure is done under general anesthesia with intubation and a ventilator to take over the patient's breathing at the beginning and end of the procedure. The surgeon performs a median sternotomy, sawing through the entire length of the breastbone, thereby providing access to the great vessels, the heart, and the coronary arteries on the surface of the heart. Various incisions and tubes are placed in the great vessels to take over the pumping of the heart and the oxygenation of blood, using a heart–lung machine in *cardiopulmonary bypass*. The heart and the breathing are stopped, and with the heart thus stilled, the surgeon can perform the placement of bypass grafts. These grafts can be saphenous veins taken from the legs. One end of a graft is sewn into the aorta, and the other end is sewn into the affected coronary artery beyond, and thus bypassing, the blockage. An alternate—and better—approach for longevity of the graft involves the use of an internal thoracic artery, of which there are two (one on each side of the chest wall). Anatomically, these are secondary branches off one of the first branches of the aorta. This branch is then taken from the attachment point in the chest wall and sewn into the affected artery beyond the blockage. Once the coronary arteries are bypassed, the heart is restarted, the patient is taken off cardiopulmonary bypass, and the chest is closed.

Compared with PCI, CABG has a higher risk (a mortality rate of 1%–25% depending on the severity of cardiac and noncardiac disease), with women having a worse outcome (Malenka et al., 2005). Hospitalization for CABG typically runs from 5 to 7 days, versus 1 night with PCI, and the recuperative period is 2 to 6 months, versus 2 to 3 days. Complications of CABG, such as postsurgical arrhythmia and infection, are not uncommon, and the long-term sequelae include prolonged cognitive deficits and depression, thought to be related to the use of the heart–lung machine. Thus, as PCI and stent technology has improved, the use of CABG has declined and will continue to do so. CABG is preferred for patients with severe left main and/or severe three-vessel coronary artery disease because it is associated with better short- and long-term outcomes for these conditions (e.g., a reduced need for recurrent procedures).

Valvular Disease

The treatment of valve disease has historically been accomplished surgically, using an open heart approach. This procedure in many ways mimics CABG; however, instead of bypassing coronary artery blockages, an incision is made in the left atrium for mitral valve replacement or in the aorta for aortic valve replacement. Either valve replacement can be accomplished with a mechanical or tissue valve. The course of recovery is similar to CABG, as are the complications.

An emerging approach to valvular disease is the use of transcatheter valve replacement, most recently being tested for replacement of a diseased aortic valve. This is a minimally invasive procedure that repairs the valve without removing the old, damaged valve. Somewhat similar to a stent placed in an artery, transcatheter aortic valve replacement delivers a collapsed replacement valve to the valve site through a catheter, where a balloon is used to expand the valve scaffold. Once the new valve is expanded, it pushes the old valve leaflets out of the way, and the tissue in the replacement valve takes over the job of regulating blood flow. Initially tested in patients with severe aortic valve disease who were not healthy enough to undergo surgery, the use is gradually being tested in healthier and younger groups to see how the outcomes compare with surgical valve replacement. In addition, a comparable approach for mitral valve replacement is now undergoing testing with older, sicker patients who are not candidates for other surgical interventions.

Cardiac Arrhythmia

The treatment of cardiac arrhythmia varies, depending on the type and source of the arrhythmia. Ventricular arrhythmias of a potentially fatal nature—those that produce severe hypotension or fibrillation—must be treated immediately with cardioversion—shock—for fast rhythms or fibrillation or with cardiac pacing for slow rhythms or bradycardias; anti-arrhythmic medications are also used. The use of shock should be well known and has been depicted countless times in movies and on TV. Perhaps less well known is the use of *implantable cardioverter defibrillators* (ICDs) for patients who are at risk of potentially fatal ventricular arrhythmias. The ICD is a sophisticated device that includes a control "box" usually implanted below the collarbone that is connected to "leads" threaded to the heart through the circulation. The box is programmed to sense the ventricular rhythm and programmed with thresholds (e.g., a slow and fast heart rate). When these thresholds are met, the device is programmed to take over pacing of the heart for several beats to return the heart to a normal rhythm. If the pacing fails to accomplish this, the device shocks the heart; the strength of each subsequent shock may be gradually increased until the rhythm returns to "normal."

Antiarrhythmic medications are designed to address key elements in the conduction of the electrical signal from the sinoatrial node and downward throughout the conduction system, along with the response of myocytes to this signal. Although these medications can be effective, they can also be difficult to tolerate and can often be accompanied by proarrhythmic side effects.

Treatment for *atrial fibrillation* (AF) depends on frequency and severity of symptoms and overall management of disease. The goals of treatment include preventing blood clots, thus lowering the risk of stroke; controlling the rate of ventricular contraction to allow the ventricles enough time to fill with blood; restoring a normal heart rhythm to allow the atria and ventricles to work together; and treating any underlying cause, such as hyperthyroidism.

Preventing blood clots from forming is probably the most important part of treating AF. The benefits of this type of treatment have been proven in multiple studies. Blood-thinning medicines to prevent blood clots include warfarin (Coumadin), dabigatran, heparin, and aspirin. People taking medicines such as warfarin must be careful of injuries that can provoke a "bleed"; they require regular checks of blood levels to ensure that the range is within acceptable parameters. Rate control is accomplished through the use of medications such as beta-blockers, CCBs, and digitalis to improve symptoms (e.g., palpitations). Medications (e.g., amiodarone, sotalol, flecainide) can also be used for rhythm control, though with risks of harm to the heart and other organs. *Cardioversion*—the use of low-energy shocks—is also used to trigger a normal rhythm. *Catheter ablation* may be used as well. In this procedure, radio wave energy is sent through a catheter threaded through the circulation to the suspected site of the conduction abnormality in the myocardium to destroy abnormal tissue that may be disrupting the normal flow of electrical signals.

Heart Failure

The treatment of heart failure (HF) is dependent on underlying causes. The main goals in therapy for chronic HF with reduced ejection fraction are

- identification and correction of underlying causes—for example, surgical repair or replacement of a "leaky" mitral valve or calcified aortic valve;
- elimination of the acute precipitating cause of symptoms in a patient who has previously been stable—for example, by treating infection or arrhythmias or removing sources of excess salt;
- management of symptoms through (a) treatment of pulmonary and systemic congestion—use of diuretic medications to rid the body of water and (b) increase of cardiac output—using vasodilating and contraction enhancing medications; and
- use of medications to modulate neurohormonal pathways and thereby slow or prevent the progression of further left ventricular dysfunction.

Because beta-blocking medications reduce the effect of SNS stimulation on the heart and thereby slow heart rate and reduce the force of contraction, their use in HF was thought to be contraindicated: With a failing ventricle it would seem that the correct thing to do is enhance contraction to maintain circulation. Yet clinical trials have shown a significant survival benefit in using these drugs for patients with HF and reduced ejection fraction (EF; López-Sendó et al., 2004). The mechanism for this effect is not fully understood but may involve the blocking of deleterious effects on myocytes that can occur with the chronic elevation in sympathetic tone that is the body's response to the failing heart. Thus, a predominant feature of modern HF care is the use of beta-blockers, along with dietary modifications to reduce sodium intake coupled with the use of diuretics to reduce fluid.

With the failing heart comes an elevated risk of potentially fatal ventricular arrhythmias, and a focus on arrhythmias, or the risk of their occurrence, has also become an important focus of HF treatment. When the EF drops below 35%, especially in the setting of acute MI, a patient becomes eligible for an ICD. A more recent advance in ICD therapy has included the use of biventricular devices that provide therapy to both ventricles—so-called *cardiac resynchronization therapy*. Although it can be life saving (i.e., the ICD prevents the heart from going into a fatal rhythm called *ventricular fibrillation*), the receipt of a shock or repeated shocks (which can sometimes be inappropriately triggered) causes some patients to develop anxiety disorders or depression. Another issue can arise in late-stage HF when a patient and family may be faced with a decision to "turn off" the ICD and end life.

Other advanced therapies can include the use of cardiac transplantation, which is limited due to the low availability of sufficiently healthy hearts to transplant, and *ventricular assist devices* (VADs), which are a form of artificial partial heart. These are mechanical pumps that are implanted between the left ventricle and aorta to support the pumping of blood from the heart and into the circulation. They are becoming increasingly sophisticated, and the number of patients both in hospital on VADs awaiting transplant and discharged to home on these devices is increasing each year. Management of these devices at home then becomes an important focus for the patient and family.

Treatment of heart failure with preserved EF is not as far advanced; indeed, this is a more recently recognized clinical presentation. The goals of therapy here are to relieve congestion and address correctable causes of stiffening (e.g., hypertension, coronary artery disease). Diuretics are often used, but cautiously so as to not affect left ventricular filling. Other standard medications do not affect morbidity and mortality.

A PSYCHOLOGIST'S ROLE

Behavioral Risk Factors

Although emotional factors—anger, hostility, depression—have been a major focus of research on psychological factors and CHD, much of incident CHD risk is attributable to what are among the "traditional risk factors," including tobacco use, diet, sedentary lifestyle, and related behaviors such as medication adherence. A great deal of research has been devoted to these lifestyle choices, the factors and constructs that contribute to the maintenance of these choices, and the best approaches to making and maintaining lifestyle changes. The psychologist has a critical role to play in these more behaviorally focused efforts. In recent years there has been a substantial reduction in the use of tobacco, in part due to the public health effort (e.g., public service announcements, billboards, media commercials, packaging of tobacco products), and these efforts have been informed by psychological research on message framing. At the same time, there has been a notable dissemination of cessation programs. These programs use behavior change principles such as motivational interviewing, goal setting, reinforcement and stimulus control, and mobilization of supportive others to accomplish the aim of smoking cessation.

Approaches that concern healthy lifestyle overall may best be epitomized by the Diabetes Prevention Program (Diabetes Prevention Program Research Group, 2002), a multicenter clinical trial that found modest weight loss accomplished through dietary changes and increased physical activity prevented or delayed the onset of Type 2 diabetes in study participants. The lifestyle intervention group received an intensive program in diet—eating less fat and fewer calories—and exercise—a total of 150 minutes a week—and behavior modification. This 16-session curriculum was taught by case managers on a one-to-one basis during the first 24 weeks after enrollment and was flexible, culturally sensitive, and individualized. Subsequent monthly individual and group sessions with case managers were designed to reinforce behavioral changes. This program, informed by sound behavioral and psychological principles, demonstrated the profound benefit of behavioral approaches to risk reduction while also showing the promise of conducting such interventions on a large scale. Since the original study, the program has been widely disseminated.

Also as noted, medication adherence, or indeed, adherence to all medical recommendations, is an essential part of treatment for heart disease. There are a number of issues that arise and interfere with adherence, including depression, as we discuss in a later chapter. Medications also can have a number of side effects that make adherence less desirable. The psychologist can play an important role as part of a larger care team to address suspected or known nonadherence. Motivational interviewing can be a powerful tool to place adherence in the context of the things that matter most to a patient. Problem-solving factors that interfere with adherence can also be useful, and this can include encouraging patients to speak frankly with their cardiologist about any side effects and whether alternate medications or dosing regimens are available. Incorporation of memory aid tools such as pillboxes, placement of medication bottles in key areas of the home, and more easily managed practices can also be a focus when working with the patient who has adherence issues.

The Stress of Managing and Treating Heart Disease

For patients with heart disease and their family members, the various and often invasive diagnostic tests and medical procedures can be an extreme source of stress. Particularly with more advanced disease, these procedures are accompanied by a remarkable degree of acute and chronic demands on the patient and family. The psychologist can play a role in supporting these individuals as they adjust to these demands in both the short and long term. This can involve some degree of short-term stress management in the form of relaxation strategies that can be helpful in the context of diagnostic tests and invasive procedures or more involved therapy concerning existential issues and coping with permanent changes to vitality and life function. Relying on pragmatic behavioral, problem-solving, and cognitive behavioral approaches can be most helpful to the patient and family, while also bringing a level of compassion and understanding informed by heart disease knowledge and understanding.

SUMMARY

This chapter completes Part I's overview of heart disease. Although this section may have been complex, it is essential for psychologists practicing in the cardiologic "space" to be sufficiently versed in the complexity of heart disease and its treatment(s) so that they can converse as true colleagues with their cardiology colleagues, while also being able to converse knowledgeably with patients, many of whom have a deep knowledge and understanding of their disease.

Part II is devoted to the common behavioral and mental health factors and conditions that can be comorbid with and affect the prognosis of heart disease, including depression, anxiety, and sleep and sexual issues, along with a focus on the family and end-of-life issues, each of which provides a context and role for the psychologist working in the cardiologic space.

TWO

COMMON CONDITIONS TREATED IN BEHAVIORAL CARDIOLOGY

4

Assessment and Treatment of Depression

Depression after a cardiac event may seem a logical, if not appropriate, response to what has likely been an unexpected, yet life-changing, incident. Indeed, depending on how depression is measured—as a diagnostic entity or a continuum of symptoms—between 15% and 35% of patients evidence some degree of depression in the days and weeks after a cardiac event. In programmatic research conducted over the past 30 years, depression has been found to be common in patients with coronary heart disease (CHD). Furthermore, it is often unrecognized and increases the risk of recurrent cardiac events and mortality. The threshold of depression severity at which risk is conferred can be quite low (e.g., a score on the Beck Depression Inventory of 10 or greater), and the pathway(s) by which depression confers risk may involve physiologic and/or behavioral mechanisms.

http://dx.doi.org/10.1037/0000070-005
Psychological Treatment of Cardiac Patients, by M. M. Burg

In several large, prospective, epidemiological studies of initially healthy individuals, a history of major depressive disorder (MDD) was associated with up to a fourfold increased risk of incident CHD, with meta-analyses showing depression to be an independent risk factor for CHD, with a relative risk of 1.64 (Rugulies, 2002). Depression is also often associated with unhealthy behaviors such as smoking, poor diet, and sedentary lifestyle (Wulsin, 2004), each of which is independently associated with incident CHD. Although these behaviors can be seen to influence the depression-associated risk, statistical analyses controlling for these additional factors have shown that depression remains a significant contributor to incident CHD. Approximately 40% of patients with CHD (chronic, stable coronary artery disease, unstable angina, or acute cardiac syndrome [ACS]) evidence clinically meaningful levels of depressive symptoms (Celano & Huffman, 2011), whereas approximately 15% to 20% meet criteria for MDD (Carney & Freedland, 2008), a rate 3 times greater than in the general population. Elevated rates of depression are also seen in patients with heart failure (HF), those receiving an implantable cardioverter defibrillator (ICD), and those who have undergone coronary artery bypass grafting (CABG); this is understandable because these clinical presentations are along the CHD continuum.

Among ACS patients with depression during hospital admission, more than half had depressive symptoms before their cardiac event, and this is also true of patients with ICDs and those admitted with an HF exacerbation. Many patients with elevated depression symptoms or who meet MDD diagnostic criteria at the time of a cardiac event no longer demonstrate meaningful elevations 3 months later, and it is uncertain whether these individuals have depression-associated risk of cardiac event recurrence or mortality. This realization may in part underlie the failure of the largest National Institutes of Health–funded depression clinical trial to date, the Enhancing Recovery in CHD Patients (ENRICHD) Trial, to demonstrate any effect of gold standard depression treatment on CHD-related outcomes (Burg & Czajkowski, 2011). Thus, more recent depression trials with patients after a cardiac event have screened for depression at the time of the event and 3 months later, enrolling and then randomizing only those patients with persistent elevation of depression symptoms (Burg et al., 2008).

WHAT LINKS DEPRESSION TO CORONARY HEART DISEASE?

The possible pathways by which depression contributes to recurrent cardiac events and early mortality in CHD patients and after ACS are many and consist of both biological and behavioral components (Carney, Freedland, Rich, & Jaffe, 1995). These include autonomic dysregulation characterized by altered autonomic activity—for example, heightened sympathetic nervous system (SNS) activity and reduced parasympathetic nervous system (PNS) activity, heightened hypothalamic–pituitary–adrenal (HPA) axis activity, endothelial dysfunction and propensity to stress-induced myocardial ischemia, elevated inflammation and associated processes, increased platelet activation, smoking and physical inactivity, and overall health risk behavior and medication nonadherence.

Altered Autonomic and Hypothalamic–Pituitary–Adrenal Axis Activity

Altered autonomic and HPA-axis activity may play a particularly important role in the connection between depression and CHD outcomes. Patients with a history of CHD exhibit a pattern of increased SNS and decreased PNS activity. This pattern of autonomic dysfunction has been associated with increased mortality in patients with prior ACS or current HF. In addition, otherwise healthy individuals with MDD demonstrate elevations in circulating catecholamines and cortisol, and the associated decrease in PNS activity and increase in SNS activity predisposes CHD patients to myocardial ischemia, ventricular tachycardia, ventricular fibrillation, and thus sudden cardiac death. Heart rate variability (HRV), a measure that describes the natural, beat-to-beat variation in the pause between heartbeats, is a direct indication of PNS activity, and reduced HRV is a strong independent predictor of mortality in both recent ACS patients and those with chronic stable CHD. Depressed patients both with and without CHD have reduced HRV, and as depression severity increases, the degree of HRV reduction does as well. Furthermore, patients with both CHD and depression have a greater degree of HRV decrease compared with patients with either alone, suggesting that the effects of depression and CHD on this indicator of PNS activity are additive. Low HRV has also been found to partially account for the effect of depression on survival after ACS in statistical models. Thus, alteration in autonomic activity that accompanies depression has a clear impact on CHD-relevant events.

Endothelial Dysfunction and Propensity for Stress-Induced Myocardial Ischemia

Endothelial dysfunction is among the earliest markers of CHD risk; this has been observed in several studies among otherwise healthy individuals with both MDD and subsyndromal levels of depression symptom severity. Depression has been associated with impaired endothelial function in those at risk of and with established CHD. Treatment of depression with selective serotonin reuptake inhibitors (SSRIs) improves endothelial function in patients with stable CHD, supporting a role for endothelial dysfunction as a link between depression and cardiac outcomes. Among patients with stable CHD, depression symptom severity is directly related to the level of endothelin-1, a biomarker involved in both endothelial dysfunction and plaque rupture. CHD patients with depression are also more likely to have a reduction in myocardial blood flow during acute psychological stress, a finding consistent with the triggering of cardiac events by sad mood. Each of these findings points to dysfunction in the normal response of the coronary arteries—down to the microvascular bed—in patients with both depression and CHD.

Inflammation

C-reactive protein (CRP), indicative of a general inflammatory state and closely linked to CHD-related outcomes, is significantly elevated in depressed patients without CHD (Carney & Freedland, 2017). These patients can also show elevations in circulating interleukin-1 and interleukin-6, each also linked to CHD-related outcomes, with findings similar for CHD patients. Among ACS patients, depression is associated with elevated CRP, though, importantly, this may be due to nonadherence to prescribed statins, which in addition to lowering cholesterol also have anti-inflammatory properties. The level of several inflammatory markers is also related to depression 2 months after a cardiac event, with patients whose first depression occurs at the time of the cardiac event showing the highest levels of inflammation. This finding raises a "chicken-or-egg" question as to whether depression "causes" inflammation and thereby contributes to CHD risk, whether CHD "causes" inflammation and thereby contributes to depression risk, or whether in depression and CHD we are looking at two sides of the same coin whereby both—depression and CHD—are essentially diseases of inflammation.

Platelet Function

Several studies have found platelet hyperreactivity in otherwise healthy depressed patients and depressed CHD patients (see Carney & Freedland, 2017). Serotonin, which is involved in depression, as evidenced by the use of SSRI antidepressant medications, is critically involved in platelet function as well, contributing to platelet aggregation in the setting of atherosclerosis. Patients with depression have elevated platelet serotonin receptor concentrations and low levels of platelet serotonin transporter. These findings combined suggest that an increase in serotonin sensitivity and impairment in the ability to remove serotonin from the circulation are present in people with depression. The platelets of depressed patients also appear to be "hyperactive"—that is, stickier and thus more likely to induce coagulation when there is a plaque rupture. This then leads to a thrombus formation and consequent cardiac event. The serotonergic and platelet dysfunction may, therefore, be an additional important pathway mediating the increased risk of CHD-relevant events in depressed patients.

Acute psychological stress also increases platelet aggregation in apparently healthy individuals and patients with CHD. Thus, after a cardiac event, when disrupted coronary plaque(s) are healing, it may be that depressed patients are at risk of recurrent events and mortality because they have a greater platelet response to stress. Specifically, the stresses experienced by the depressed patient as they try to adjust in the immediate and intermediate post-ACS context may cause the formation of new thrombus at the site of the initial ACS event, thereby leading to another ACS event.

Behavioral Factors

Several behavioral factors may interact with the previously described underlying biological substrate, including adherence to medical recommendations—for example, for increasing physical activity, maintaining a healthy diet, stopping smoking, and taking prescribed medications that are designed to impair platelet function and mitigate inflammation. Patients with mild to moderate depression symptom severity after a cardiac event are less likely to make prescribed changes to lifestyle, and those with a diagnosis of MDD and/or dysthymia are the least adherent to recommended changes in diet and exercise and to taking medications as prescribed. Studies that have found significant associations between depression and these risk factors have also found that depression predicts CHD morbidity and mortality independently (Hippisley-Cox, Fielding, & Pringle, 1998) and that it can potentiate the effects of these risk factors on CHD morbidity and mortality (Anda et al., 1993).

In the Heart and Soul Study (Whooley et al., 2008), depressed CHD patients had 50% more adverse CHD events over several years of follow-up, but this risk was no longer elevated after adjustment for behavioral adherence factors. Other research has suggested that the role of inflammation as a linkage between depression and CHD may be related in part to physical activity (Elderon & Whooley, 2013). Depressed individuals engage in less physical activity, and lower activity is associated with inflammation. Indeed, engagement in regular physical activity is a good method for reducing inflammatory states. In the large Whitehall II Cohort Study (Hamer & Molloy, 2009), physically active individuals had persistently lower inflammatory markers. Together, these findings suggest that physical activity and inflammation may combine to explain the link between depression and CHD.

Nonadherence to cardiovascular medications after a cardiac event is strongly linked with poor medical outcomes, contributing to a 3 times higher recurrence risk and greater than two- to threefold elevated risk of major adverse events and mortality in patients with stable CHD (Biondi-Zoccai et al., 2006; Ho et al., 2006). Among patients with persistent depression after a cardiac event, medication adherence can be quite low; however, those patients whose depression improves in the months after the event generally return to higher levels of medication adherence. In the current age of post-ACS and chronic CHD treatment, medication adherence may be a particularly relevant behavioral factor linking depression to CHD outcomes. This may especially be the case for patients who undergo percutaneous coronary interventions with drug-eluting stent because a failure to take medications (e.g., Plavix or clopidogrel) as prescribed carries with it the high risk of a catastrophic cardiac event at the site of the stent.

ASSESSING DEPRESSION

The diagnostic criteria for major depression include depressed mood and loss of interest in usually pleasurable activities (anhedonia), with at least five out of seven additional symptoms present nearly every day (changes in sleep, changes in appetite or weight change, psychomotor changes, fatigue or loss of energy, feelings of guilt or worthlessness, diminished concentration, suicidality). A minor depression diagnosis requires fewer symptoms beyond the hallmark depressed mood and anhedonia. As mentioned earlier, many of the symptoms in the depression constellation mirror those experienced secondary to having a cardiac event or having HF. This can complicate the assessment of depression in CHD patients.

Interview Assessment

To address the issues inherent in depression assessment among CHD patients, the ENRICHD investigators developed the Depression Interview and Structured Hamilton (DISH; Freedland et al., 2002), which is now widely used for assessing major depression and depression severity in clinical trials with CHD patients. These studies require a highly efficient interview to minimize burden. Furthermore, in contrast to studies or clinical situations in which patients self-identify because they recognize they are experiencing mood problems, CHD patients rarely self-identify and are unaccustomed to discussing potential emotional issues. Thus, it is essential that depression assessment is accomplished in a flexible, sensitive manner that fosters the development of rapport, trust, and self-disclosure. DISH-informed assessment works well in a clinical setting.

The assessment begins with open-ended questions to build rapport and encourage disclosure. Examples include "Would you mind telling me about your heart attack (or recent cardiac event or hospitalization)?" and "What's this whole experience been like for you?" (Freedland et al., 2002, p. 898). These questions communicate the concern of the interviewer, allow the patient to talk about the cardiac event and hospital experience, and provide an entrée for the next section that concerns current depression symptoms. This section includes the probes needed to identify the presence of diagnostic criteria for MDD. The wording of probes depends on patients' descriptions of their symptoms. For example, some patients deny feeling "sad" or "depressed" but admit to feeling "down" or "blue." The burden is on the clinician to judge whether the patient's terms are synonymous with the MDD criteria. The flexibility inherent in the DISH structure allows it to be easily modified to fit the medical context of the patient group being assessed for depression.

Questionnaire Assessment

Patient Health Questionnaire

The broad implementation of depression assessment among patients with CHD has for practical purposes required the development and testing of shorter screening tools (Thombs, Ziegelstein, & Whooley, 2008). The two-item Patient Health Questionnaire (PHQ-2) addresses the cardinal depression symptoms of depressed mood and anhedonia and takes only moments to complete; a "yes" response to one or both questions is 90% sensitive but only 69% specific for MDD in CHD patients, making it useful for ruling out depression. The nine-item version (PHQ-9) with a threshold score of 10 or higher is highly diagnostic of MDD. Given the utility of these instruments, their combined use in a two-step process for screening CHD patients has been incorporated into recommendations issued by the American Heart Association (AHA; Lichtman et al., 2008). In a test of this approach, a positive screen, even in the absence of MDD, was found to predict recurrent cardiovascular events (Elderon, Smolderen, Na, & Whooley, 2011), thereby indicating that the large-scale implementation of this two-step screening may be useful for targeting treatment.

There has been some concern about the AHA recommendations, largely because there is no evidence to support routine screening for depression among CHD patients—that is, there is no evidence that doing so will be cost-effective or will improve outcomes. There have also been concerns about patient misdiagnosis and unnecessary stigma and the lack of providers to whom patients with a positive screen can be referred. These combined concerns have led some to suggest that the AHA recommendations be submitted to a clinical trial. When depression screening is paired with a program for treating the depressed CHD patient, there is evidence that outcomes are better: improved adherence, reduced CHD symptoms, reduced cardiac events, improved risk factor profile (K. W. Davidson et al., 2010). Thus, systematic screening might best be implemented in settings where treatment is available.

Beck Depression Inventory

The Beck Depression Inventory (BDI; A. T. Beck, Steer, & Brown, 1996), originally developed to track progress in cognitive therapy for depression, is another instrument that has been broadly used in studies of depression in CHD patients. This self-report measure has over 20 items grouped by diagnostic symptom (e.g., depressed mood, anhedonia, feelings of guilt, sadness, discouragement, crying, changes in appetite, sleep difficulties, suicidal ideation), and the patient chooses a response that indicates a level of severity for each item. Overall scores have accepted anchors for depression severity (mild, moderate, severe), though research on depression and CHD commonly uses a score of 10 or greater because this is associated with poorer prognosis.

Hamilton Depression Rating Scale

The Hamilton Rating Scale for Depression (HAM-D; Hedlund & Viewig, 1979) is a 21-item questionnaire that, like the BDI, is "tagged" to the symptoms and signs of MDD, while also providing a metric of symptom severity. It is thus used to provide an assessment of MDD, as a measure of symptom severity, and as a guide to evaluate the effects of treatment and recovery. Although it can be administered in a self-report manner, it is usually administered in the context of a clinical interview, and it is used in this manner as part of the DISH. The HAM-D has been used in several studies of patients with CHD, though most often as an indicator of treatment effects.

Hospital Anxiety and Depression Scale

The Hospital Anxiety and Depression Scale (HADS; Zigmond & Snaith, 1983) is another self-report instrument that can also be administered in the context of a clinical interview. It consists of 14 items, seven that concern depression and seven that concern anxiety. The HADS can, therefore, be particularly useful for assessing these two often comorbid conditions. The HADS was created as a treatment outcome measure that specifically avoided a focus on somatic symptoms (e.g., fatigue, sleep disruption), and it can, therefore, be particularly useful when assessing depression in medical patient groups such as those with CHD, where somatic symptoms often accompany the medical disorder.

TREATING DEPRESSION IN PEOPLE WITH CORONARY HEART DISEASE

Depression interventions for CHD patients have received a great deal of attention, particularly for immediate and recent post-ACS patients and, more recently, HF patients. This research has focused beyond reducing depression and has aimed at determining whether the delivery of effective, depression-reducing treatments improves medical outcomes. The selection of interventions in these clinical trials has been guided by the depression treatment literature that has involved otherwise healthy individuals, with the investigations testing pharmacologic agents, particularly SSRIs, or evidence-based psychotherapies, including cognitive therapy, interpersonal therapy, and problem-solving therapy.

Pharmacotherapy

The Sertraline Antidepressant Heart Attack Randomized Trial (SADHART; Glassman et al., 2002) was an early trial designed to test the safety of SSRI medications for patients with CHD, focusing on the medication sertraline. The reason this small trial first focused on safety was that earlier antidepressant medication classes were found to increase risk of CHD-relevant events (e.g., potentially fatal arrhythmia). At the time of SADHART, SSRIs were new.

The relatively small SADHART found sertraline to be safe, with no untoward effects compared with placebo on left ventricular ejection fraction, blood pressure, heart rate, cardiac arrhythmias, or any electrocardiogram parameter. There was a modest improvement in depression—both diagnosis and Hamilton Rating Scale for Depression score—and although it was not statistically significant, there was a lower incidence of major adverse cardiac events at the end of the 24-week treatment period. A secondary analysis of data collected as part of a sub-study found evidence that the plasma levels of sertraline in patients randomized to receive treatment were directly related to improvement in platelet and endothelial biomarkers, indicating a pathway by which SSRI medication might work to improve post-ACS outcomes—that is, by improving endothelial health and reducing the propensity of platelets to aggregate. A more recent randomized trial testing the safety of sertraline for treating depression in patients with HF found this antidepressant medication to be safe for this patient group (Jiang et al., 2011). In this trial, although treatment was not associated with a greater reduction in depression or improvement in cardiovascular status compared with placebo, remission of depression was associated with better HF-related outcomes.

In the Canadian Cardiac Randomized Evaluation of Antidepressant and Psychotherapy Efficacy (CREATE) Trial (Lespérance et al., 2007), patients with CHD, defined as prior ACS or coronary revascularization, and comorbid MDD were randomized in a complex factorial design to a 12-week course of the SSRI citalopram versus placebo and/or interpersonal psychotherapy (IPT). All study participants also received clinical management. The focus of this trial was on depression, not medical outcomes. In this trial, patients randomized to citalopram had a significantly greater reduction in depression symptom severity at the end of the 12-week treatment period compared with patients on placebo, though the effect size was moderate at best. There was also no benefit on depression severity for IPT versus clinical management.

The Myocardial Infarction and Depression-Intervention Trial (de Jonge et al., 2007) was another test of antidepressant medication (mirtazapine) for postmyocardial infarction patients with depression. This trial randomized 331 patients with MDD at 0, 3, 6, 9, and 12 months after myocardial infarction (MI) to either antidepressant treatment ($n = 209$) or care as usual ($n = 122$). Of those randomized to treatment, 45 received no treatment (due to refusal); 94 were randomized to mirtazapine versus placebo, and of these, 46 were switched to citalopram because they remained depressed while receiving the initial medication; and 40 received nonpharmacologic depression treatment. No differences in depression or cardiac event rate were observed for patients who received any treatment compared with controls (14% for intervention, 13% for controls) up to 18 months after their MI, whereas secondary analyses found a lower cardiac event rate for responders.

Psychological Interventions

The ENRICHD Trial was the first multicenter randomized clinical trial that was large enough ($n = 2{,}481$) to test the effects of depression treatment on a primary endpoint of recurrent MI and mortality in patients with MDD after MI (Writing Committee for the ENRICHD Investigators, 2003). For this trial, individual cognitive therapy for depression as developed and disseminated by J. S. Beck (1995) was chosen for the intervention, and the focus of treatment was remission of depression. This individual therapy was augmented by group-based psychotherapy that included both depression remission strategies and stress-reduction strategies, though, for logistical reasons, only about one third of patients randomized to treatment participated in group sessions. Patients not on a predetermined improvement trajectory were offered augmentation with sertraline, and treatment was delivered for up to 6 months after initiation. The improvement in depression symptom severity at 6 months (the end of treatment) was modest compared with usual cardiologic care; however, there were no effects on medical outcomes. Furthermore, the effect of treatment on depression was substantially reduced at 12-month follow-up. However, the investigators described the troubling sign that minority women assigned to the treatment group had worse medical outcomes. This mirrored an earlier finding in a study conducted in Montreal of "case management" for distress in CHD patients (Frasure-Smith et al., 1997). In that study it was found that among women, those who did not show improvement in the weeks immediately after initiation of treatment had worse outcomes, demonstrating the importance of delivering an effective treatment. A smaller clinical trial of cognitive therapy for depression in patients with HF (Freedland, Carney, Rich, Steinmeyer, & Rubin, 2015) found the intervention to be effective for depression remission but not for congestive heart failure self-care or physical functioning, though there were additional benefits for anxiety and fatigue reduction, social functioning, and health-related quality of life.

The disappointing results of the ENRICHD Trial led the investigators to consider the factors that might have contributed to the modest effect of treatment on depression and the lack of any effect on medical outcomes. First, they observed "spontaneous remission" among patients randomized to usual care within months of their cardiac event. Therefore, the cardiac event rate may have been substantially lower than expected in the usual care group; any effect that depression might have had was eliminated. This pointed to the likelihood that many patients who "look" like they have depression in the days after an ACS event may only be experiencing adjustment issues and therefore not at depression-associated risk of recurrent ACS and mortality. The take-home message is that psychologists have to engage in "watchful waiting" before launching depression treatment. If what looks like depression remits in 1 to 3 months, there is no need to treat; if, however, depression persists, treatment should be initiated. The ENRICHD investigators also identified issues of patient engagement with the intervention. As noted earlier, CHD patients with depression do not identify themselves as such, attributing any depression symptoms they have to their heart disease. It can, therefore, be difficult to engage them in a therapy such as cognitive therapy, especially considering the degree to which the focus of therapy sessions is on the automatic thoughts that can be depressogenic, compared with focusing on behavioral activation, which can make more sense for the CHD patient.

A promising set of smaller ($N = 150–157$) multicenter clinical trials—the Coronary Patients Evaluation Study (COPES; K. W. Davidson et al., 2010) and the Comparison of Depression Interventions after Acute Coronary Syndrome (CODIACS) Vanguard Trial (K. W. Davidson et al., 2013)—took these lessons from the ENRICHD experience. In each of these trials, there was a 3-month period of watchful waiting after a cardiac event, and only those patients with persistent depression, both at the time of their event and 3 months later, were randomized. In addition, a diagnosis of MDD was not necessary to meet eligibility. Rather, a threshold score on the BDI (≥ 10) associated with cardiac recurrence and mortality was used. These trials also addressed the issue of patient engagement by using brief problem-solving therapy and SSRI medication in a 6-month patient preference, stepped-care approach that is usually acceptable to medical patients with depression. In this approach, the patient chooses between problem-solving therapy or SSRI medication. Progress in therapy is reviewed at 2-month intervals, and if reduction in depression symptoms is not sufficiently evident, treatment is enhanced. In both trials, ACS patients had significant reduction in depression symptoms compared with usual care, and patients expressed high satisfaction with the treatment. In the COPES trial, treatment was also associated with a reduced risk of death or hospitalization for MI or unstable angina at the end of the 6-month treatment period. This effect did not persist after treatment ceased, however. It may be that depression among CHD patients should be considered a chronic disease that requires ongoing surveillance after symptoms remit and reengagement with booster sessions when symptoms reemerge. Psychotherapy approaches that include self-surveillance—perhaps with a smartphone app that reports symptom elevations to the patient's provider—may be worth testing.

As noted earlier, several professional organizations have recently published recommendations for stepped depression assessment post-ACS and provision of treatment to patients who meet designated thresholds, despite the slim evidence for either screening for, or treating, depression in these patients. The ability to mount effective psychotherapy treatments is hampered by logistical issues, leaving the easier prescription of SSRI antidepressant medications—again with a slim evidence base. Furthermore, SSRIs carry bleeding risk—an issue for patients on multiple antiplatelet agents—and may have little benefit for the mild or moderate depression severity often seen in cardiac patients. Depression is a diagnostic syndrome characterized by a constellation of symptoms that fall into distinct groupings (e.g., cognitive, somatic, affective), and it remains unclear which grouping is "cardio-toxic." Future depression clinical trials powered to major adverse cardiac event outcomes are needed to ascertain the best approach to this important issue.

DEPRESSION IN THE CLINICAL CONTEXT

Depression Subtypes

A review of the diagnostic criteria for depression quickly reveals that depression is a syndrome characterized by a constellation of symptoms. These symptoms include affective, cognitive, behavioral, and somatic elements. A diagnosis can be made when any of several different combinations of these elements is present in a patient. This is also true when considering depression symptom severity, whether the severity is above or below the threshold for a diagnosis, raising important questions concerning depression in CHD patients, the relationship of depression to CHD-related prognosis, and the pathways linking depression to prognosis. Thus, when assessing depression in chronic CHD patients or in those who have recently experienced a cardiac event, it becomes essential to identify the patient's unique depression features and then match the treatment to the patient and his or her unique presentation subtype.

Anhedonia may be a unique feature related to CHD prognosis because those with anhedonia may be at high risk of nonadherence to medication, exercise prescription, and overall medical recommendations. Thus, when considering treatment, it may be sufficient to use the behavioral activation component of cognitive therapy as a way to "jump-start" and reestablish the behavior-reinforcement relationship. Yet, it is essential to include a focus on adherence, including to medication, health risk behavior change, and engagement in cardiac rehabilitation as aspects of the reengagement with activities and events that are a part of behavioral activation.

The timing of depression in relation to acute cardiac events or cardiac exacerbations may also be associated with better or worse CHD outcomes. As described in the diagnostic criteria, depression is a recurring and remitting disease with first onset typically in the setting of a major life event early in adulthood. In the description particularly of the ENRICHD Trial, the issue of timing in relation to the cardiac event had implications for distinguishing between a true depression—which carries prognostic risk—and an adjustment disorder, which apparently does not. Watchful waiting with repeat assessment may, therefore, be the best approach for these patients. Timing can also be important in regard to whether the patient is experiencing a depression recurrence. For example, both CREATE and SADHART found SSRIs had greater benefit for recurrent depression versus new onset depression.

Many patients with depression in the context of a cardiac event report no prior history even when interviewed by skilled diagnosticians using structured interview formats. This raises questions as to whether this "incident depression" has unique underlying pathophysiology and whether this unique pathophysiology has a distinctly cardio-toxic element. For example, incident depression may reflect a highly malignant inflammatory process that is affecting key brain regions. It remains to be tested whether anti-inflammatory treatments address this presentation.

Symptom classes (e.g., cognitive vs. somatic) and treatment resistance have also been discussed as important features that should inform treatment. Given that somatic symptoms of depression are often seen in CHD patients—particularly after a cardiac event—and that these symptoms may be evidence of compromised cardiovascular function rather than depression, one should not be surprised if this symptom class is predictive of CHD prognosis. The use of multivariate statistical modeling that controls for CHD severity can go just so far, and thus it can be difficult to address this issue.

Treatment resistance in depression may also be an important feature for predicting outcomes after cardiac events, as found in ENRICHD, though efforts to address treatment resistance—for example, using a stepped care approach in which treatment is intensified—have not been subject to rigorous testing. The COPES and CODIACS trials took an approach comparable to this; however, as with previous efforts, treatment was confined to a 6-month window once initiated.

Integrating Depression and Cardiac Care

Although both large and small clinical trials have been directed at the question of whether treating depression after ACS reduces recurrence and mortality risk, this question remains largely unanswered. Several large trials have failed to show benefit (cf. Writing Committee for the ENRICHD Investigators, 2003), whereas a few small trials have shown promise (K. W. Davidson et al., 2010, 2013). Two trials have even shown a disturbing "signal" that the psychotherapy intervention was harmful to minority women (cf. Frasure-Smith et al., 1997). Yet, despite the absence of a clear, evidence-based treatment path, several national and international professional organizations have published consensus statements and guidelines for screening and referral for treatment of cardiac patients with depression (cf. Lichtman et al., 2008).

Screening for depression in the primary care setting is increasingly a part of standard care. Although this creates the possibility of improving depression and reducing CHD events, it can only be useful and effective when treatment options are available and the support needed to ensure patient engagement is in place. In the absence of this structure, screening is at best futile and at worst harmful. The U.S. Preventive Services Task Force specifically recommended having an identified depression care manager working in concert with a supervising psychiatrist; however, other mental health providers—especially psychologists specifically trained to work with cardiac populations—can oversee and facilitate the needed patient activation, follow-up, symptom monitoring, and treatment intensification as needed (Siu & U.S. Preventive Services Task Force, 2016).

Screening in the specialist's office (e.g., the cardiologist's office) or at the time of cardiac diagnostic testing or intervention can similarly be useful to identify the patient with previously unrecognized depression or unrecognized depression recurrence. Again, although there appears to be "value added," it remains essential to have in place a referral and support system to ensure proper follow-through by the patient and continuous monitoring by the health care system. As integrated care expands and takes hold and the reach of the accountable care organization experiment grows, each point of contact for any patient becomes an opportunity to screen and evaluate for depression and then refer for and manage subsequent treatment. Regardless of the setting in which screening, assessment, and treatment occur, it is the nature of depression that treatment decisions can be complex, and treatment must be individually tailored and results monitored.

The integration of mental and physical health care can be accomplished with success for patient outcomes and satisfaction with a team-based, collaborative care approach, as demonstrated with cardiac patients in COPES and CODIACS. Exercise interventions can also be highly effective for improving depression in cardiac populations and are standard components of cardiac rehabilitation. Achieving and maintaining motivation can be difficult in this comorbid group. Emerging technologies—particularly smartphone-based apps and text messaging—are being developed and tested as supportive adjuncts for depression treatment. These can be particularly useful to support behavioral activation and health risk behavior change efforts in depressed patients with CHD, with additional technologies now focusing on monitoring medication adherence and providing real-time information to providers so as to address nonadherence as needed.

CLINICAL VIGNETTE

Mrs. Anderson,[1] a 72-year-old woman, experienced complications following CABG surgery and spent 10 weeks in a rehabilitation facility. After returning home, she initially resisted participation in a cardiac rehabilitation program but agreed after much urging from her family members. During the intake, she endorsed many symptoms of depressed mood on the BDI. On further questioning, she stated she had been depressed since her hospital discharge. She reported that her mood before hospitalization had been good, and she recalled no prior depressive episodes. She expressed shock that she had nearly died following her surgery and was distressed that she had no memory of approximately one week of her hospitalization. She questioned whether her somatic symptoms (fatigue, insomnia, weight loss) were due to her mood or her heart disease but with discussion agreed that multiple factors were likely contributors. She ruminated following her return home as to whether she should be "getting her affairs in order." She gradually became an active participant in cardiac rehabilitation, noting that it was helpful to talk to other people who were also coping with cardiac recovery.

After a few weeks in cardiac rehabilitation, she accepted a referral for her depression. She attended 45-minute psychotherapy sessions in conjunction with cardiac rehabilitation. Psychotherapy took a cognitive therapy approach that supported and encouraged her efforts toward "behavioral activation" and her return to previously enjoyable activities with church groups, family, and friends. The therapy also was supportive of Mrs. Anderson in addressing her feelings about the severity of her cardiac disease, the upheaval of adjusting to life with heart disease, and her grief at the realization that her life could have ended with no apparent

[1] The details of the case studies appearing in this volume have been changed to preserve the anonymity of the individuals involved.

warning. With a heightened appreciation of her mortality, she was able to focus on the things that were important to her. Her symptoms of depression remitted within 14 weeks. Mrs. Anderson stated that the combination of the physical activity and peer support in cardiac rehabilitation, the opportunity to process her emotions in psychotherapy, and the passage of time were all helpful in her recovery.

This vignette illustrates that many patients might not avail themselves of mental health services if they believe their symptoms to be a natural consequence of cardiac disease. Psychological adjustment can progress more quickly with focused attention on the emotions associated with diagnosis and treatment of serious illness.

SUMMARY

Depression increases the risk of cardiac event recurrence and early mortality in patients with CHD. Several pathways have been identified as possible links between depression and CHD prognosis, and the failure to identify a "smoking gun" may reflect the syndromal nature of depression, whereby different presentations are related to different pathways, all reaching the same bad ending. Standard depression treatments have largely been shown to be safe; however, the effect on medical prognosis remains to be demonstrated, notwithstanding two small trials of integrated care. The "integrated depression care" approach may have its greatest likelihood for implementation within the larger integration of care across disciplines that is occurring nationwide, including within accountable care organizations.

5

Assessment and Treatment of Anxiety

Although feelings of anxiety and frank anxiety disorders can be highly prevalent among cardiac patients, anxiety as a prognostic factor has not garnered the attention depression has. Prospective studies of initially healthy individuals indicate that there is an increased risk of sudden death and myocardial infarction (MI) in patients with panic disorder, and the physiological correlates of anxiety, particularly the cardiovascular concomitants, can implicitly be assumed to increase coronary heart disease (CHD) risk, mediated by stress reactivity in the autonomic and hypothalamic–pituitary–adrenal (HPA) axis pathways. This chapter describes the comorbidity of anxiety and heart disease, the link between anxiety and CHD-related outcomes, the possible pathways underlying this linkage, the anxiety assessment methods used for CHD patients, and the treatment literature.

http://dx.doi.org/10.1037/0000070-006
Psychological Treatment of Cardiac Patients, by M. M. Burg

ANXIETY BASICS

Anxiety is a common experience that includes cognitive and affective elements, a sense of fear and unpredictability, and apprehension about the future. It can be viewed as a normative reaction to a range of situations or as a dispositional tendency to react under conditions of uncertainty. Anxiety crosses the threshold into a disorder when experienced frequently, intensely, and under inappropriate circumstances, leading to feelings of helplessness and impaired psychological and physical functioning (Lader & Marks, 1973). In contrast to depression, *anxiety disorder* is an umbrella term for a set of disorders that includes generalized anxiety disorder (GAD), panic disorder, and phobias. Almost 30% of adults will have an anxiety disorder in their lifetime (lifetime prevalence of GAD is 5.7%, panic disorder 4.7%, specific phobia 12.5%, and social phobia 12.1%). Posttraumatic stress disorder (PTSD) is part of the *Diagnostic and Statistical Manual of Mental Disorders* (5th ed.; American Psychiatric Association, 2013) category of trauma or stressor-related disorders, and recent research has begun to elaborate a specific manifestation of PTSD that occurs as a consequence of a cardiac event (discussed later). Although the research on depression and CHD has revealed a particular symptom severity threshold for adverse CHD-related risk, the nature of anxiety as an appropriate set of responses under given conditions makes the identification of a similar threshold difficult.

Despite the fact that anxiety can be a normative response, research has suggested that chronic anxiety increases incident CHD risk among initially healthy individuals, even when controlling for standard risk factors. In early studies of initially healthy men followed prospectively, high-anxiety symptoms increased the risk of fatal CHD significantly, a finding that remained consistent in later studies. In a meta-analysis of these studies, anxiety carried a pooled hazard ratio of 1.26 to 1.48 for incident CHD, cardiac mortality, and nonfatal MI (Roest, Martens, de Jonge, & Denollet, 2010). No differences in this effect were found according to the type of anxiety or gender, and overall, the strength of these effects persists in more recent studies. Taken together, this research indicates that, like depression, anxiety contributes to cardiac risk and associated mortality.

Anxiety is also a common experience for patients with chronic CHD, with the prevalence up to 25%; for those who have experienced a cardiac event, the prevalence can be over 70%. Although anxiety is normative during and in the days after any cardiac event, persistence as the patient recovers can hinder adaptation and physical recovery. Anxiety contributes to reduced quality of life and interferes with both rehabilitation and the ability to integrate the information necessary to make needed lifestyle changes and maintain a medication regimen. Patients with persistent anxiety after a cardiac event return to work more slowly or less often and have more difficulty resuming sexual activity. This constellation has been termed *cardiac invalidism*, which describes disability after acute coronary syndrome (ACS) that is not accounted for by the severity of CHD (Sullivan, LaCroix, Spertus, & Hecht, 2000).

POTENTIAL PATHWAYS LINKING ANXIETY AND HEART DISEASE

As with depression, several pathways have been proposed as linkages between anxiety and cardiac disease, and these include both physiological and behavioral factors.

Physiological Factors

States of anxiety and the general psychological stress thereby engendered can lead to changes in autonomic tone, such as an increase in sympathetic nervous system (SNS) activity and a decrease in parasympathetic nervous system activity, particularly cardiac vagal control. This is manifested by such things as an increase in circulating levels of catecholamines—epinephrine and norepinephrine—and a decrease in heart rate variability. There is also an increase in HPA-axis activity—an increase in circulating cortisol and a change in the associated diurnal pattern. This is true for both otherwise healthy individuals and patients with CHD. As described in earlier chapters, this pattern over time can lead to endothelial damage and the establishment of atherosclerotic plaque. There is also a greater reactivity to stressors, particularly anxiety-provoking events experienced routinely, and this can lead to an increase in resting heart rate, altered baroreflex sensitivity, and elevated risk of arrhythmia. Among patients with implantable cardioverter defibrillators (ICDs), a bout of anxiety during the day can provoke potentially fatal arrhythmias, especially for those with chronic anxiety, and these experiences can trigger atrial fibrillation in patients with this disorder. Thus, together, these autonomic and HPA-axis effects may increase the risk of incident CHD through the promotion of atherosclerosis, while lowering the threshold for myocardial ischemia, cardiac arrhythmias, and sudden cardiac death.

Through these autonomic and HPA-axis pathways, high levels of anxiety may contribute to platelet aggregation and thrombus formation as well. Again, as noted earlier, epinephrine and norepinephrine cause—among other things—an increase in platelet aggregation and, thus, together with effects on autonomic tone, can set the stage for plaque rupture leading to a cardiac event. A review paper by von Känel, Mills, Fainman, and Dimsdale (2001) concluded that patients with CHD who are prone to greater reactivity under conditions of daily stress—much like patients with anxiety—are at risk of acute events due to these pathways. These effects may be further enhanced when anxiety is—as is often the case—comorbid with depression.

There is also evidence that extreme emotional states, such as acute anxiety episodes, can trigger a cardiac event in patients without coronary obstruction. This has been termed *broken-heart syndrome*, *left ventricular apical ballooning syndrome*, and *takotsubo cardiomyopathy* (Wittstein et al., 2005). The typical patient presents with symptoms of ACS and on diagnostic imaging is found to have significantly impaired left ventricular function, although no coronary obstruction. The types of triggering events have included the unexpected death of a loved one or other tragic news, fear of choking, fear of public speaking, and fear of a medical procedure. The mechanisms underlying this syndrome appear to involve a profound level of SNS activity and secretion of catecholamines—a form of catecholamine poisoning, which at the cellular level results in the stunning of cardiac myocytes. The syndrome usually resolves within days, with no lasting cardiac impairment. Yet, patients who experience this cardiac syndrome have also experienced a profound major life event as a precipitant and thus may benefit from attention to their overall adjustment and their underlying psychological risk of acute reactions to major life events.

Behavioral Factors

Anxiety is associated with several health risk behaviors that can contribute to incident CHD and poor prognosis after a cardiac event. People with anxiety are more likely to smoke cigarettes, consume excess alcohol, have a sedentary approach to physical activity, and eat a less healthy diet. Patients with anxiety after a cardiac event are also less likely to complete cardiac rehabilitation and are more likely to be nonadherent to their medication regimens. This scenario is again similar to what is seen in depression, though the reasons may be different. For example, for patients with anxiety after a cardiac event, the cardiac rehabilitation setting may be perceived as threatening. These individuals are likely to be more sensitized to bodily signals such as the increase in heart rate that accompanies physical exertion, and thus when they note the increase in their heart rate, their sense of anxiety increases as well. Such a patient presents a particular challenge for staff at these programs. It is a part of cardiac rehabilitation for patients to learn that they can safely exert themselves and have an increase in heart rate within a safe range. The patient is taught to monitor their heart rate during exercise. But for the anxious patient, monitoring of heart rate may have the opposite effect, thereby increasing anxiety. This patient may require more attention than other patients, attention that staff may not be able to give. Thus, as with the depressed patient, the anxious patient is at risk of dropout.

ASSESSING ANXIETY

Anxiety in CHD patients may best be assessed using a stepped approach, starting with brief self-report screening and moving to full interview-based assessment guided by initial responses. A number of brief instruments can be useful for ascertaining symptom severity.

The PRIME-MD (Spitzer et al., 1994) is a self-report questionnaire consisting of 26 questions about the presence of symptoms and signs during the preceding month. It serves as an initial screen for five groups of mental health issues, including anxiety. Because the questions are self-report, diagnoses of an anxiety disorder or symptom severity must be verified, taking into account patient understanding of the questions, along with other relevant information from patients, their families, or other sources. An Anxiety Severity Index is calculated by assigning scores of 0, 1, 2, and 3 to the response categories of *not at all*, *several days*, *more than half the days*, and *nearly every day* for the seven anxiety items, respectively. The total score ranges from 0 to 21. Scores of 5, 10, and 15 represent cutoff points for mild, moderate, and severe anxiety, respectively. Though designed primarily as a screening and severity measure for GAD, this index also has moderately good validity for panic disorder, social anxiety disorder, and PTSD. When screening an individual for any anxiety disorder, a recommended cutoff point for further evaluation is a score of 10 or greater.

The General Anxiety Disorder-7 (GAD-7; Spitzer, Kroenke, Williams, & Löwe, 2006) is a more recently developed self-report tool for assessing anxiety that can also be used as an initial screening tool. The seven items of the scale address anxiety symptoms, including feelings of nervousness or anxiousness, worry, restlessness, irritability or annoyance, and unspecified or ungrounded fear and difficulty relaxing. As with the PRIME-MD, the patient endorses items along a continuum from *not at all* (0), *several days* (1), *more than half the days* (2), and *nearly every day* (3), and the total anxiety score is the sum of all items. In addition to this scoring, the patient is asked to indicate for any endorsed items how difficult these problems have made it for the patient to do his or her work, take care of things at home, or get along with other people. Scores of 10 or greater have 89% specificity and 82% sensitivity for a diagnosis of GAD. The developers of the GAD-7 noted the high comorbidity of anxiety and depressive disorders and the high correlation between depressive and anxiety measures, and indeed, scores on the eight-item Patient Health Questionnaire (PHQ) and GAD-7 are highly correlated. However, factor analysis confirmed that anxiety assessed by the GAD-7 was distinct from depression assessed by the PHQ, with many patients scoring high on the GAD-7 not having high depression symptom severity and patients with high anxiety symptom severity having corresponding high impairment in multiple domains of functional status.

The Spielberger State–Trait Anxiety Inventory (STAI; Spielberger, Gorsuch, Lushene, Vagg, & Jacobs, 1983) is a commonly used self-report measure of trait and state anxiety that has been widely used for research concerning anxiety in medical populations. It has a sixth-grade reading level and can be a useful instrument for distinguishing anxiety from depression. It consists of 20 items for assessing trait and state anxiety. Each item is scored on a 4-point scale (from *almost never* to *almost always*) indicating the extent to which the patient experiences the described anxiety indicator. State items include "I am tense; I am worried" and "I feel calm; I feel secure." Trait items include "I worry too much over something that really doesn't matter" and "I am content; I am a steady person" (American Psychological Association, 2017b). The instructions for the trait and the state items differ in the time frame the patient is asked to consider when thinking about the questions. The score for anxiety is the sum of item scores, with some items being reverse scored (e.g., "I feel calm"), and higher scores indicate greater anxiety. This instrument is often preferred because the items do not focus on a specific aspect of anxiety, but rather comprise a wider sampling of anxiety symptoms. The inclusion of items that are reverse scored addresses the likelihood of a patient engaging in an automatic response pattern without attending to the individual items.

The Beck Anxiety Inventory (BAI; A. T. Beck, Epstein, Brown, & Steer, 1988) is a 21-question self-report inventory that is used for measuring the severity of anxiety symptoms. For each item, patients are asked to indicate on a 4-point scale how much they were bothered by the symptom during the preceding week. Thus, this scale is best considered a measure of acute or state anxiety. Given the nature of the 21 items, the BAI has a greater focus on somatic symptoms that occur with panic disorder.

The Hospital Anxiety and Depression Scale (HADS; Zigmond & Snaith, 1983) was described in the previous chapter on depression. Briefly, the HADS consists of seven items that assess depression and anxiety, and thus it can be particularly useful for assessing these comorbid conditions. It was created as an instrument that did not include somatic items, making it highly useful for assessing these dimensions with CHD patients.

The Cardiac Anxiety Questionnaire (CAQ; Eifert et al., 2000) is an 18-item self-report questionnaire that was developed to assess the condition of *heart-focused anxiety* (HFA), the fear of cardiac-related stimuli and sensations because of their perceived negative consequences. Although this anxiety condition and the associated distress can occur in the absence of CHD, it can be particularly disabling for patients diagnosed with CHD, especially those who have experienced a cardiac event. Items reflect the three factors (I—*worry* about chest and heart sensations, II—*avoidance* of activities believed to elicit cardiac symptoms, III—*attention* to the heart and monitoring of cardiac activity) assessed by the scale and are endorsed by the patient along a Likert scale from 0 (*never*) to 4 (*always*). A total score is computed as the mean score for each of the 18 items, and subscale scores are computed similarly, ensuring that the total and subscale scores can be more directly and easily compared. Higher scores indicate greater HFA. Given the specific focus of this assessment tool, it can be particularly useful for distinguishing HFA from generalized anxiety and can thus help focus treatments designed to improve the quality of life and life engagement after a cardiac event.

The ICD Concerns Questionnaire (ICDC; Frizelle, Lewin, Kaye, & Moniz-Cook, 2006) is a 20-item self-report questionnaire that was developed to measure the extent and severity of concerns experienced by patients with an ICD. Two factors—perceived limitations because of having an ICD (e.g., limitations to exercise, activity, physical intimacy, and work due to fear of provoking an ICD shock) and device-specific concerns (e.g., pain or symptoms with shock, battery or device malfunction, lack of control over shock, impact on future)—are assessed, with items endorsed along a Likert scale from 0 (*not at all*) to 4 (*very much so*). Higher scores indicate greater concern. The ICDC can be used clinically by health care providers involved in ICD patient care to identify specific concerns and target intervention accordingly.

Self-report screening instruments are useful for their ease of administration. They can be completed before the office visit, and the responses of patients can be incorporated into the assessment in the context of the typical office encounter. More in-depth questioning and more structured interviewing in person are then warranted, as indicated by responses to questions, and the direction taken during this more in-depth interview should be guided by the screening questions, given the diverse nature of anxiety disorders (e.g., generalized anxiety, panic, agoraphobia, specific phobia). Such an interview and discussion can be undertaken in a manner that normalizes the patient experience, thereby helping to reduce any sense of stigma the patient may be experiencing.

A challenge to proper screening and identification of anxiety in patients with CHD is posed by the overlap of anxiety and cardiac symptoms, including palpitations, elevated heart rate, and chest discomfort. Panic disorder can be a particular issue: One quarter of patients presenting to the emergency department with chest pain may have panic disorder. Women are particularly at risk of being labeled as "worried well," even though it is known that the symptoms women experience during a cardiac event can be atypical, and even chest pain in the absence of coronary occlusion increases the risk of ACS and early mortality. Thus, careful questioning and differential diagnosis are critical.

PSYCHOLOGICAL TREATMENT OF ANXIETY

No clinical trials have specifically tested whether treating anxiety in CHD patients affects ACS recurrence, mortality, or revascularization, though there have been a number of smaller trials of what one might broadly term *psychosocial interventions* for this population (see the Cochrane reviews: Baumeister, Hutter, & Bengel, 2011; Whalley et al., 2011). The interventions in these studies largely included multiple components (e.g., relaxation training, goal setting, behavioral risk reduction, cognitive reframing), and the participants included patients with (and without) anxiety, depression, chronic stress, and/or distress. Findings demonstrated small-to-moderate effects on depression and/or anxiety. On the basis of these findings it is clear that much remains to be accomplished to establish an evidence base for how best to address anxiety in the context of heart disease.

What Components of Anxiety Are Most Toxic?

As with depression, anxiety is a condition with affective, cognitive, somatic, and behavioral components, each of which may uniquely contribute to incident CHD risk and subsequent prognosis. *Rumination*, the uncontrollable repetitive and intrusive thinking about an often-distressing topic, is a cognitive component that can promote distress and depression and repeated and sustained activation of autonomic and HPA axis stress response systems, making it a potentially important mediator between anxiety and CHD. Rumination has been the focus of considerable research, and reviews have suggested that these effects, along with effects on sleep, may uniquely contribute to increased risk of incident CHD (Ruiz, Hutchinson, & Terrill, 2008). Panic is another aspect of anxiety that may increase CHD risk, here too likely due to the repeated activation of stress response systems. Cognitive and behavioral avoidance associated with anxiety after a major cardiac event may be involved in failures concerning health-risk behavior change and medication adherence; I discuss this aspect of anxiety next as concerns posttraumatic stress secondary to ACS.

Treatment Approaches

Anxiety interventions are often similar to depression interventions, as might be expected given the comorbidity and symptom overlap. Yet, anxiety interventions contain some unique components that include relaxation-based elements (diaphragmatic breathing, imagery, mindfulness meditation). People who have experienced shock from an ICD are examples of a subpopulation of cardiac patients who may benefit from a relaxation-based intervention. Cardiac patients who have experienced shock are at heightened risk to develop PTSD. PTSD is a disorder that develops as a consequence of exposure to traumas such as natural disasters, sexual assault, automobile accidents, and combat. PTSD is also found in the general cardiac population. Its estimated prevalence as a consequence of a cardiac event is 12%, varying from 4% to 32% across studies, depending on PTSD assessment methods (Burg & Soufer, 2016). Demographic factors associated with PTSD include being younger, being female, belonging to an ethnic minority, and having low socioeconomic status. The course of PTSD after a cardiac event can be variable, with some patients showing remission, others showing persistence, and still others showing late onset. PTSD after a cardiac event increases 1-year cardiovascular readmission and both early cardiac recurrence and mortality up to 50%, with patients who report high levels of reexperiencing symptom cluster (e.g., intrusive thoughts, nightmares) having the highest risk (Burg & Soufer, 2016). In a meta-analysis, a positive screen for PTSD caused by a cardiac event doubled the risk of adverse medical outcomes (Edmondson et al., 2012). Patient experiences in the emergency department environment appear to be involved in PTSD onset and thus may provide an opportunity to prevent PTSD and improve outcomes. Similarly, the reexperiencing symptom cluster may require both cognitive behavior therapy for insomnia for better outcomes. Given that reexperiencing can lead to behavioral avoidance, a focus on associated reminders of the cardiac event may provide an avenue for improved outcomes in the clinical population. During exercise cardiac rehabilitation, providers place a specific focus on putting the patient at ease with the increase in heart rate while exercising. The issues of safety in activity and training in skills to address stress reactivity—both cognitive/emotional and physiological—become paramount for the cardiac patient with anxiety.

How Should the Clinician Proceed?

Clinical psychologists working independently or in the context of a cardiac rehabilitation program or integrated care setting should be aware that many patients perceive mental health treatment to be stigmatizing. During the initial interview, the clinician should ascertain whether the symptoms being experienced are (a) lifelong versus recent, with the onset of CHD; (b) distinguishable between symptoms of anxiety and CHD progression and exacerbation; and (c) distinguishable between the different anxiety presentations (e.g., generalized, phobic, panic) if indeed anxiety is present. The challenge is to distinguish anxiety symptoms from cardiac symptoms (e.g., palpitations, elevated heart rate, chest discomfort). Panic disorder can be particularly challenging and lead to unnecessary emergency department visits because symptoms are often believed by a patient to mean he or she is having a heart attack. As described earlier, women present a particular challenge, given the atypical nature of their CHD presentation. Therefore, careful assessment is critical.

Once anxiety is identified, treatment becomes essential for patients to return to their prior level of functioning. A stepped-care approach can be as useful for anxiety as it appears to be for depression. With milder cases of anxiety, reassurance, exercises to promote functionality and increase confidence, and training in relaxation and problem-solving techniques are usually effective. Attention to adherence, whether to cardiac rehabilitation, exercise routines, medications, and/or lifestyle changes, should also be included. Motivational interviewing techniques help promote a greater degree of patient autonomy and choice, and personal goal setting can be useful in these efforts. Ongoing monitoring of adherence as treatment progresses is essential.

Patients with more severe levels of anxiety and distress require further treatment. It is helpful if behavioral care can be provided in the same medical setting and in the context of a coordinated visit. This sends a holistic message to patients (i.e., of a consonance between mind and body) and can increase their confidence in the system of care. It can also reduce barriers to receipt of care. When medication is indicated, SSRI antidepressants are frequently used for efficacy with anxiety and safety with cardiac populations. In all cases, ongoing monitoring and follow-up are advised.

A treatment algorithm developed by Pozuelo and colleagues (2009) for assessing and addressing depression can also be useful for anxiety. The algorithm starts with a brief screen for the issue; applying this to anxiety one might use the GAD-7 because it was specifically designed for this purpose, though the HADS may be more useful with a cardiac population for whom cardiac symptoms mirror those of both depression and anxiety. If the patient "screens in" for anxiety, further interviews can help determine the nature of the anxiety and the specificity to the cardiac situation in relation to prior history. If the patient has no prior history and has only recently experienced a cardiac event or exacerbation, reassurance and watchful waiting may be sufficient. Regardless, some discussion of treatment options and approaches is the next step in the algorithm. Because the patient likely did not seek out treatment for anxiety, this discussion may best be accomplished with an initial focus on how the anxiety experience is affecting quality of life—in particular, impact on work, home, social relations, and outside activities. In this way, reluctant patients can be helped to understand the potential benefits to addressing their anxiety. If treatment is indicated and agreed on, the choices are reviewed; Pozuelo et al. recommended either SSRI medication for up to 9 months with a gradual taper thereafter or brief (three to six sessions) psychotherapy (e.g., cognitive behavioral therapy). Continued monitoring of symptoms throughout treatment and thereafter for up to 6 weeks as indicated helps determine the effectiveness of treatment and whether further treatment efforts are warranted.

OUTSTANDING ISSUES

Comorbidity of Anxiety and Depression

Anxiety disorders and depressive disorders frequently co-occur, raising potential issues of confounding; because there is considerable overlap in symptom presentation, statistical control is often not adequate. Some have argued that it may be more fruitful to consider that together depression and anxiety are more reflective of general distress, which studies have shown contributes to CHD risk (Strik, Denollet, Lousberg, & Honig, 2003). The literature remains mixed, and thus for the time being it may be best to assess each separately and consider the overall symptom cluster when making decisions about how to proceed with treatment of the CHD patient.

Gender

Women are at an approximately twofold higher risk of anxiety disorders compared with men, and this appears true internationally for both developed and developing countries, regardless of the specific anxiety classification. Studies examining the relationship of anxiety to CHD provide little evidence of an effect for gender. Because incident CHD occurs on average 10 years later for women than for men—likely due to the protective effects of estrogen before menopause—the effects of anxiety as a chronic condition may be masked. Once CHD is established, however, anxiety may be involved in the unique features of this disease for women, including a higher prevalence of coronary microvascular disease and a greater degree of functional impairment after a cardiac event. Furthermore, women with occult CHD are often underdiagnosed or misdiagnosed (e.g., as having an "anxiety problem"). They are sent home from the emergency department when they present with vague complaints that are consistent with and attributed to "anxiety" by staff (e.g., palpitations, chest "discomfort," and elevated heart rate). This is a consequence in part of both the known higher prevalence of anxiety among women and the differences in symptoms of ischemia between men and women. Yet women with this "nonspecific chest pain" have double the risk of ACS and related mortality.

Women with CHD are also more likely to live alone, which in the context of anxiety and distress can both increase recurrent cardiac event risk and make them resistant to treatment, as seen in the ENRICHD trials (Burg & Czajkowski, 2011; see also Chapter 4, this volume) and in a telephone-delivered, collaborative care postcoronary artery bypass grafting treatment trial (Rollman et al., 2009). These studies highlight the need for clinical approaches that address the unique needs of women with CHD. A group-based treatment specifically for women with CHD was undertaken in a recent trial conducted in Sweden, which found an almost threefold protective effect of the stress-reduction intervention over 7 years of follow-up (Orth-Gomér et al., 2009).

CLINICAL VIGNETTE

This clinical vignette highlights the manifestation of anxiety in the context of progressive cardiac disease. Multiple methods of anxiety intervention are illustrated for the same patient.

Mr. Lopez was referred to Dr. Bloom, a clinical psychologist working with both the cardiac rehabilitation and arrhythmia clinics. Mr. Lopez had a failing heart and had experienced three MIs before the age of 60. An ICD had been implanted approximately 2 years before the referral. The patient stated that he had recovered well after each of his earlier cardiac events and had lived with no difficulty with the ICD for the first 18 months. However, during a family vacation, the ICD fired multiple times, and Mr. Lopez experienced a great deal of anxiety related to this trauma. He reported that he had become afraid to be alone and fearful that the ICD would fire unexpectedly. He had become preoccupied with this worry and found it difficult to focus at work. He avoided using the restroom due to fear of being alone and avoided activities that he previously enjoyed. Dr. Bloom conducted a clinical interview. In addition, he had the patient complete standardized questions concerning experience with his ICD: the Florida Shock Anxiety Scale, a 10-item measure of ICD-specific feared stimuli and avoidance behaviors that includes items such as, "I am scared to exercise because it may increase my heart rate and cause my device to fire" (Kuhl, Dixit, Walker, Conti, & Sears, 2006).

As a result of this assessment, Dr. Bloom determined that the patient had an acute stress reaction. Intervention focused on specific fears related to the patient's preoccupation with the possibility that the ICD might fire again. Cognitive behavior therapy (CBT) incorporated systematic desensitization and exposure to decrease Mr. Lopez's avoidance behaviors and cognitive reframing to think of the ICD as a lifesaving device. The therapist provided support and education in the context of CBT, and Mr. Lopez's anxiety diminished over approximately six sessions. This vignette illustrates that cardiac anxiety often stems from appropriate concern and responds well to interventions that pinpoint specific fears and behaviors.

SUMMARY

Anxiety may increase the risk of CHD, with evidence that it can also contribute to cardiac recurrence and mortality. Although having feelings of anxiety is a normal reaction to a cardiac event, the feelings can persist and promote poor adherence to the very interventions that improve outcomes, and this can particularly be the case for individuals with a history of anxiety, those with comorbid depression, and those who typically engage in ruminative thinking about events that might or could happen. Women can be particularly affected. There are effective treatments for anxiety, but research on the effects of these treatments for improving CHD outcomes has been limited. For clinicians, it may at this time be most useful to consider the impact of anxiety on a patient's overall functioning. With a stepped-care approach to both assessment and treatment, clinicians can be of greatest use in providing needed care for the anxious cardiac patient. Doing so in the context of overall care through an integrated care framework can be most beneficial for the patient.

6

Assessment and Treatment of Sleep Dysregulation

The importance of sleep as a factor that contributes to incident coronary heart disease (CHD), to CHD progression, and to prognosis after a cardiac event has been recognized only recently, and the assessment of sleep in the context of large observational studies is an emerging literature. Furthermore, sleep is often linked to CHD-related comorbidities (and the medications used to treat them), including hypertension, diabetes, heart failure, hyperlipidemia, obesity, and mental health conditions including depression, anxiety, chronic stress, and posttraumatic stress disorder (PTSD). Nonetheless, the evidence linking sleep dysregulation to CHD outcomes is compelling, with some calling for sleep to be included among the standard risk factors used to predict CHD. In this chapter, I summarize the literature on the comorbidity of sleep dysregulation with CHD and discuss the nature and impact of fatigue in the context of CHD. I describe methods used for assessment of sleep dysregulation and

http://dx.doi.org/10.1037/0000070-007
Psychological Treatment of Cardiac Patients, by M. M. Burg

provide an overview of the most effective and recommended treatments for disrupted sleep.

NORMAL SLEEP

Sleep, which involves regular disengagement from the environment, reduced sensory input, and decreased energy expenditure, is observed in all animal species. It consists of three states—wakefulness, rapid eye movement (REM) sleep, and non-REM (NREM) sleep—though assessment and descriptions of sleep focus on four stages (NREM sleep has two stages). Each stage has unique characteristics.

Approximately four to five NREM and REM cycles occur during nighttime sleep, with each successive REM episode gradually getting longer. NREM sleep is characterized by altered autonomic tone—decreased sympathetic nervous system (SNS) activity, and increased parasympathetic system activity—and cardiovascular function—decreased stroke volume, heart rate, respiration, peripheral vascular resistance, and blood pressure; body temperature falls as well. Other body processes increase, including immune function, hormone release (growth factor and cortisol), and protein synthesis. REM sleep is accompanied by sympathetic and overall brain activity that is similar to that observed when awake. Each REM cycle has a tonic state that is interspersed with phasic states, with their characteristic "rapid eye movements." These states have distinct autonomic nervous system and cardiovascular profiles that can change rapidly, with sudden bursts of SNS activity that occur in phasic REM sleep, in part linked to changes in muscle tone. There is an accompanying increase in heart rate and blood pressure to levels seen during wakefulness.

There is considerable variation in the amount of sleep a healthy person requires, and the average amount that people get has changed as technology has progressed. For example, before electricity became available, it is estimated that people slept approximately 9 to 10 hours per night, but with electricity and, more recently, the spread of Internet access, a normal amount of sleep is now considered 6.5 to just under 9 hours per night. This fact highlights the role of light in the regulation of the sleep–wake cycle.

SLEEP AND RISK OF INCIDENT CORONARY HEART DISEASE

It is estimated that as few as one third of adults in the United States get the recommended amount of sleep, with another one third getting fewer than 6.5 hours (Centers for Disease Control and Prevention, 2009, 2011). This essential sleep deprivation—and, over time, accumulated sleep debt—has been linked to metabolic disorder and CHD (Gallicchio & Laesan, 2009). The Nurses' Health Study of 71,617 initially healthy female participants found that short self-reported sleep duration was independently associated with an increased risk of cardiac events over 10 years of observation (Ayas et al., 2003). Insufficient sleep also increases risk of diabetes and hypertension, whereas not getting enough sleep and getting too much sleep are associated with obesity, CHD, stroke, and diabetes, independent of sex, age, race and ethnicity, and education.

In a population-based cohort study of over 20,000 initially healthy adults conducted in the Netherlands, short versus normal sleep duration was independently associated with a 23% elevated risk of incident CHD over 12 years of follow-up (Hoevenaar-Blom, Spijkerman, Kromhout, van den Berg, & Verschuren, 2011). A Norwegian cohort study of over 50,000 adults found more specifically that, compared with people who never experience sleep issues, difficulty initiating sleep almost every night was associated with a 45% increased risk of myocardial infarction (MI), difficulty maintaining sleep almost every night was associated with a 30% increased risk, and feelings of nonrestorative sleep more than once a week were associated with a 27% increased risk (Laugsand, Vatten, Platou, & Janszky, 2011). Combined, there was a dose-dependent association between the number of these symptoms and MI risk, and an editorial response to the paper suggested that sleep disturbances should be added to the list of modifiable risk factors for incident CHD (Redline & Foody, 2011). A meta-analysis of 15 studies with a combined sample of over 470,000 participants with follow-up ranging from 6.9 to 25 years reported that short duration of sleep was associated with a greater risk of developing or dying of CHD (48% elevated risk) or stroke (15% elevated risk), whereas long duration of sleep was also associated with a greater risk of these outcomes (Cappuccio, Cooper, D'Elia, Strazzullo, & Miller, 2011). Overall, these findings indicate that both short and long sleep increase risk of CHD and related mortality.

DISORDERS OF SLEEP

Lack of sleep or reduced sleep duration is common and can be by choice, due to personal constraints such as work or family commitments, or due to the circumstances of illness such as hospitalization in noisy environments. Fragmented or poor quality sleep can be a consequence of medical issues (e.g., pain), psychological issues (e.g., anxiety), medications (antidepressants, beta-blockers, narcotics, glucocorticoids), cardiac devices (pacemakers), and acute interventions (e.g., breathing support in an intensive care unit). Common sleep problems include

- insomnia or hypersomnia,
- sleep-related movement disorders (e.g., restless legs syndrome), and
- sleep-related breathing disorders (e.g., obstructive sleep apnea).

Insomnia is defined as difficulty initiating and/or maintaining sleep. Initiation should occur within 30 minutes of an effort to initiate sleep (e.g., going to bed). Most people experience some degree of short-term insomnia. Insomnia can result from *poor sleep hygiene*, a term used to describe practices that negatively affect sleep, which include the lack of a regular sleep routine (e.g., time in and out of bed), ingestions (e.g., caffeine, alcohol, nicotine) within several hours of sleep, and sleep-distracting activities (e.g., watching TV in bed). Insomnia can also result from excessive worry and perseverative cognition or rumination and can accompany mood disorders. When insomnia is prolonged (i.e., more than 6 months in duration), it is defined as chronic and requires attention.

Hypersomnia (daytime drowsiness or excessive sleep) in the absence of disrupted nighttime sleep may be due to a mood disorder, sleep-disordered breathing, or medications. Depression can be accompanied by sleep that is not restorative, leaving the individual feeling sleepy throughout the day.

With depression, delayed onset of REM sleep can occur. A confounding issue associated with treatment of mood disorders is that antidepressants can cause drowsiness and periodic limb movements, which fragment sleep.

Restless legs syndrome is characterized by an unpleasant sensation in the legs when seated or lying in bed, accompanied by an urge to move the legs; that movement provides a brief reduction in the sensation. There is a strong circadian aspect, which can be used to measure severity. For example, it is classified as severe if the onset is as early as before dinnertime, modest if the onset occurs after dinnertime but before bedtime, and mild if the onset is after the person has gone to bed. The etiology of restless leg syndrome is unclear, and there is some suggestion of a familial link. Treatment can involve iron therapy and dopamine agonists.

Obstructive sleep apnea (OSA) is a primary sleep disorder characterized by repeat episodes during sleep when an individual ceases breathing due to a transient obstruction in the upper airway during inspiration (i.e., intake of breath), with each episode of obstruction lasting between 20 and 40 seconds. The person may snore and experience frequent arousals and sleep fragmentation and loss, accompanied by chronic sleepiness and drowsiness. The prevalence of OSA is estimated at 24% among men and 9% among women, making it a common problem. The causes of OSA include the increase in soft tissue around the neck that accompanies obesity, age, and decreased muscle tone in the throat, which can be secondary to alcohol use.

With each OSA episode there is an increase in SNS activity, accompanied by peripheral vasoconstriction, increased cardiac output, and thus a dramatic increase in arterial blood pressure. There is also an increase in platelet activation, and thus a prothrombotic state, and a notable bradycardia that can increase the risk of a cardiac arrhythmia. Together, these autonomic, hemodynamic, circulatory, and myocardial effects can lead to chronic CHD and can trigger episodes of cardiac ischemia, acute cardiac syndrome events, and stroke. Left untreated, OSA will eventually lead to glucose intolerance and overt diabetes, increased endothelin and decreased nitric oxide bioavailability, endothelial dysfunction, increases in systemic inflammation, and incident hypertension, congestive heart failure, and mortality.

ASSESSMENT OF SLEEP

Polysomnography

Polysomnography is a comprehensive assessment approach that includes the recording of several bodily functions and the changes in these functions while the person sleeps. It is performed in a sleep laboratory during a person's normal sleep hours (e.g., at night or daytime for shift workers). In the typical arrangement, the patient reports to the sleep lab in the early evening; labs are located in dedicated hospital units, medical offices, or hotels. The patient is introduced to the sleep setting (e.g., bedroom) and fitted with various electrodes and sensors that are wired to a central box so that multiple channels of data can be recorded during sleep; the box is connected to a computer. A sleep technician is in attendance to monitor the patient during the study, observing sleep activity and the computer display of data in real time. The test is completed, and the patient is discharged home the next morning except when assessment of daytime sleepiness is called for.

Recent advances in technology allow for the conduct of polysomnography assessment in a person's home, using ambulatory measurement tools that incorporate storage of digital information for later analysis. Many people experience difficulty sleeping in new locations, so the expansion of polysomnography to the home can provide for a more accurate assessment. The physiological indices that are typically assessed during polysomnography include brain activity (electroencephalogram), eye movements (electrooculogram), muscle activity (electromyogram), heart rate and rhythm (electrocardiogram), breathing function (respiratory airflow and effort), and pulse oximetry. The comprehensive approach entailed in polysomnography makes it the gold standard for diagnosing narcolepsy, idiopathic hypersomnia, periodic limb movement disorder, REM behavior disorder, parasomnias, sleep apnea, and disorders of sleep architecture (sleep stages).

Actigraphy

As an alternative to polysomnography, *actigraphy* can be used to measure cycles of activity and rest, including sleep and sleep quality. The actigraph is similar to many commercially available wrist-worn devices that have come on the market in recent years, though those used for assessment of sleep problems are more sensitive and have been validated in controlled experimental studies. When used to assess sleep, an actigraph is worn each day for 1 to 2 weeks. The most recent devices also include light sensors and are thereby able to determine aspects of the sleep environment. By using an actigraph, it is possible to assess how active a person is during his or her self-designated sleep time and thus determine the actual hours of sleep per night and the quality of sleep during each episode of sleep. Actigraphy also provides a reliable estimate of movement and light, from which circadian rhythm can be estimated.

Questionnaire Assessment

It is also possible to use self-report questionnaires to assess dimensions of sleep. Perhaps the most used questionnaire is the Pittsburgh Sleep Quality Index (PSQI; Buysse, Reynolds, Monk, Berman, & Kupfer, 1989). The PSQI consists of 10 items. Items 1 to 4 concern usual bedtime and awake time, typical amount of time to fall asleep, and typical number of hours of sleep; each of these questions is placed in a time frame of the past month. Item 5 has nine components that concern specific sleep difficulties (e.g., difficulty getting to sleep, difficulty staying asleep, feeling too hot or too cold, pain, bad dreams), and the patient is asked to indicate the frequency of the problem over the past month (not at all, less than once a week, one to two times a week, three or more times a week). Other items inquire into the use of sleep medication, difficulty staying awake during daytime activities, and reports from the patient's bedroom partner—if there is such a partner—of symptoms that are consistent with OSA. The PSQI provides for scoring of sleep along multiple parameters, including subjective sleep quality; sleep latency, duration, and efficiency; sleep disturbances; and daytime dysfunction.

TREATMENT OF DISORDERED SLEEP

Sleep Hygiene

Sleep hygiene is a set of practices developed almost 40 years ago to address mild to moderate insomnia. It is based on the notion that sleep is a natural part of existence and that the body "knows" how to sleep. Behavioral practices and environmental context interfere with this natural ability, and thus sleep hygiene is designed to return the body to the natural condition to reestablish the normal pattern. The practices focus on the reestablishment of a sleep routine when it has been disrupted and involve both behavior and the sleep environment. The specific recommendations include the following:

- Establish a regular sleep schedule. This form of "stimulus control" includes going to bed at the same time each night and getting up at the same time each morning. It also involves largely doing away with naps. It furthermore involves using the bed only for sleep or sexual activity and not for reading, listening to music or commentary, or watching TV. Last, an additional instruction is to not stay in bed for more than 10 to 15 minutes without sleeping—that is, if sleep does not come in 10 to 15 minutes after going to bed or if awakened in the middle of the night, one should not remain in bed for more than 10 to 15 minutes if sleep does not reoccur. If these conditions do arise, the person is encouraged to leave the bed and sit in a chair in the dark until he or she feels drowsy, at which time he or she should return to bed.
- Avoid physical and mental exercise in the hours before the set bedtime. Although regular exercise can promote good sleep, it is important that the body and mind be in a restful state in the hours leading up to bed. This is also true for stimulating mental activities. Each leaves the body and/or mind in an activated state that is not conducive to sleep.
- Avoid caffeine, tobacco, and alcohol in the hours before bedtime. The effects of caffeine can last for many hours, causing difficulties in initiating sleep and subsequently fragmenting sleep. Thus, the patient is encouraged to avoid caffeinated beverages of any kind for up to 12 hours before bedtime. Nicotine, like caffeine, is a stimulant and thus should

also be avoided in the hours before bedtime. Last, although alcohol is typically thought of as a relaxant or depressant, it has disruptive effects on sleep and can cause fragmentation and nonrestful sleep. Thus, it too should be avoided in the hours before sleep.

- It is recommended that the sleep environment is quiet, dark, and cool. Noises, light, and uncomfortable temperatures can disrupt continuous sleep. Associated recommendations include having comfortable bedding and eliminating a visible bedroom clock, although it is important to set an alarm in order to get out of bed the same time each morning.

Research on the effectiveness of sleep hygiene recommendations for mild-to-moderate insomnia is equivocal. Sleep hygiene studies have typically used different sets of recommendations, and a recent review found the only weak evidence that this approach improves sleep quality outside clinical settings (Irish, Kline, Gunn, Buysse, & Hall, 2015). The strongest support is for the negative effects of noisy sleep environments, alcohol consumption in the hours before sleep, engaging in mentally difficult tasks before sleep, and trying too hard to fall asleep. Recommendations regarding the effects of napping depend on the length and timing of napping and cumulative nightly sleep in recent days. Nonetheless, there is support showing positive sleep outcomes for people who follow more than one sleep hygiene recommendation (Hauri, 2011), and sleep hygiene recommendations can be useful for patients with depression who may be taking naps during the day, consuming alcohol near bedtime, and consuming large amounts of caffeine during the day.

Cognitive Behavior Therapy for Insomnia

Cognitive behavior therapy for insomnia (CBT-I) aims to improve sleep habits and behaviors by identifying and changing thoughts and behaviors that are impeding the ability to sleep or sleep well. This approach contains much if not all of the recommendations that accompany good sleep hygiene and expands on these by including a focus on additional factors that may be contributing to poor sleep. The first step in CBT-I is to identify causes of insomnia, taking into account the possible factors that may be affecting sleep. The patient is encouraged to keep a sleep diary for several weeks, recording such things as time in and out of bed, activities before bed, number of awakenings and factors that interfere with sleep. This helps identify behavior, thoughts, and emotions; stress-related factors; and other variables that are affecting sleep and sleep quality. The CBT-I steps then implemented include standard sleep hygiene with stimulus control and sleep restriction, adding relaxation training, and cognitive therapy:

- *Relaxation training* includes a collection of practices such as imagery and diaphragmatic breathing that can help promote a relaxed physical and mental state in the moments before sleep or when awakening during the night. The patient is instructed in the preferred practice and encouraged to use these in relation to sleep.
- In contrast to typical cognitive therapy, as applied to sleep problems, *cognitive therapy* entails education as a means of addressing dysfunctional beliefs and attitudes specifically about sleep. Through the therapeutic interchange, the patient's beliefs and attitudes about sleep are identified, and the logical bases for these are then questioned Socratically, so as to identify underlying flaws in logic. For example, many patients believe that if they do not get enough sleep, they will be tired the entire following day. They then try to conserve energy by not moving around or by taking a nap, which can then exacerbate the problem. Worry is also common among people with disrupted sleep. Worry and rumination are addressed through the use of a thought record, providing opportunities for using cognitive therapy approaches to address the specific worries individually (see also Chapter 5's discussion of CHD-related anxiety).

Although the evidence supporting sleep hygiene alone is equivocal, studies have shown improvement in insomnia for patients who receive sleep hygiene in combination with CBT-I. This includes patients with depression: A recent study showed that augmenting antidepressant medication with CBT-I in patients improved sleep and reduced depression severity (Manber et al., 2008). Studies have also shown that CBT-I improves sleep and overall functioning for patients with PTSD (Talbot et al., 2014). Other studies have suggested that CBT-I in combination with *imagery rehearsal therapy*, a technique that involves recalling a recurrent nightmare, writing it down, modifying the dream in a positive way, and rehearsing the new dream to create a cognitive shift, improves PTSD-related sleep problems.

Snoring and Obstructive Sleep Apnea

OSA and the associated symptom of snoring present a distinct set of issues that compromise sleep. Nonetheless, a first step is to identify and promote improvement in sleep hygiene–related factors. This is followed by efforts directed toward additional lifestyle factors that contribute to obesity. Changes in sleep posture and the bed are also suggested, including avoiding sleeping with a flexed neck, having patients sleep on their side rather than their back, and raising the head of the bed several inches. Having patients sew something (e.g., a ball) into the back of their pajama tops can keep them from sleeping on their back.

A second step can involve surgical correction of anatomic problems, as indicated. This includes adenotonsillectomy, correcting a chronically deviated nasal septum, and maxillomandibular advancement, excision of the tongue base, and refashioning of the uvula. Dental devices to either advance the jaw or widen the maxilla can also be useful.

More common for the adult with OSA is pneumatically splinting open the upper airway with continuous positive airway pressure (CPAP) delivered through a face mask. The mask is anatomically fitted to the individual patient. The continuous pressure of air being delivered to the mask works to keep the airway open. Adherence to the CPAP treatment can create issues. Many patients object to the face mask, finding it restricting or "suffocating"; this can be a particular problem for patients with comorbid PTSD. There are also the restrictions in movement associated with the mask and hoses, the noise produced by the CPAP machine, and the regular need to clean all the equipment to prevent bacterial infection. Each of these can produce nonadherence. Supportive psychotherapy in concert with motivational interviewing techniques can be helpful, along with directed problem-solving efforts, for improving adherence. Emerging devices that include upper airway muscle pacemakers, expiratory nasal valves, and negative-pressure oral devices show promise but remain to be fully tested in large clinical trials.

CLINICAL VIGNETTE

On meeting a psychologist for evaluation, Ms. Taylor stated that she was grateful to be alive. She had experienced an MI and had been transported by ambulance to the hospital. She underwent open-heart surgery and returned home after a 6-day hospitalization. She noted that neither her father, who had died of lung cancer in his early 50s, nor her mother, who died from chronic obstructive pulmonary disease at age 70, had ever been diagnosed with heart problems. At age 61, Ms. Taylor had not expected to be diagnosed with heart disease. She described her sleep pattern before hospitalization as normal: She had previously slept approximately 7 hours per night. Following her discharge from the hospital, she was able to fall asleep without difficulty but woke up each night and could not fall back asleep. She estimated that she slept about 4.5 to 5 hours a night. She felt fatigued during the day. She had been diagnosed with OSA approximately 2 years before the MI and had been prescribed a CPAP at that time but had not complied with using it. She found the CPAP suffocating and stated that she felt she could not be close to her husband when wearing it.

Psychological intervention incorporated education about the importance of having an oxygenated blood supply. The diagnosis of CHD increased Ms. Taylor's motivation to take steps to improve her health and to try the CPAP again. She agreed to track her sleep pattern and use the CPAP. Her husband attended one session of therapy and provided reassurance that he was not adversely affected by her use of the CPAP. Supportive psychotherapy helped Ms. Taylor process her feelings related to adjustment to heart disease. Cognitive techniques helped the patient to disrupt her tendency to ruminate and worry at night. This case illustrates that many underlying factors contribute to sleep difficulty, and behavioral intervention usually addresses a broad range of potential contributors.

SUMMARY

Sleep dysregulation is common in the cardiac population and manifests most often as insomnia. Insomnia is one of the most common reasons that cardiac patients to seek behavioral intervention. Insomnia responds well to psychological intervention but requires comprehensive assessment and a multipronged approach to intervention. Poor compliance with using a CPAP is also common among people with heart disease, and psychological intervention can be effective to improve adherence in this regard.

7

Assessment and Treatment of Sexual Dysfunction

Issues with sexual function are highly prevalent among men and women with coronary heart disease (CHD) and have a significant impact on the quality of life for patients and their partners. For males, in particular, impairment in sexual functioning (e.g., erectile dysfunction [ED]) is often an accompaniment of key risk factors for CHD, including hypertension and diabetes, but it can also be an indication of underlying endothelial dysfunction and associated CHD risk. After an acute coronary syndrome (ACS) event or in the context of advanced cardiac disease (e.g., CHD, implantable cardioverter defibrillator [ICD]), concerns related to the exertion associated with sexual activity can create further issues in this domain. Although a good bit of attention has been devoted to these issues for male patients and their partners, much less is known about how this issue affects female CHD patients. In this chapter, I describe

http://dx.doi.org/10.1037/0000070-008
Psychological Treatment of Cardiac Patients, by M. M. Burg

the range of issues associated with sexual function in CHD patients and review methods for assessment. I discuss recommendations for how to address sexual functioning among CHD patients and emphasize outstanding questions.

SEXUAL FUNCTIONING AMONG CARDIAC PATIENTS

There is a clear realization among those who provide cardiologic care of the intrinsic relationship between CHD and sexual functioning. This includes the shared underlying pathophysiology between erectile dysfunction and CHD and the concern among patients and providers that engaging in sexual activity can trigger cardiac symptoms and ACS events. In addition, some cardiac medications (e.g., beta-blockers) provoke problems with sexual functioning, increasing the likelihood that the patient will become nonadherent to the medication regimen. Moreover, the popularity of oral agents (e.g., Viagra, Cialis) and the potentially fatal interaction that can occur between these agents and organic nitrates makes them clearly contraindicated for patients on nitrates, which can raise issues of medication adherence and, in the absence of frank discussions with providers, can also lead to inadvertent use of these agents without the knowledge of the providers. Last, after an acute cardiac event of any kind, patients and their partners are often fearful of engaging in sexual activity, either due to fear of causing another cardiac event or, for the patient with an ICD, fear of causing a shock.

Given the importance of sexual functioning for optimal quality of life, the complications presented by CHD, the potential issues related to medication therapy for ED in this group, and the warranted and unwarranted fears, it is essential that within the overall delivery of cardiac-related care, sexual function be included as an element of equal importance to standard factors of lifestyle and medication management. Indeed, the absence of this approach leaves patients and their partners unnecessarily fearful and at risk of medication nonadherence or the inadvertent mixing of drugs that can result in catastrophic outcomes.

ASSESSMENT FOR SEXUAL ISSUES IN PATIENTS WITH CORONARY HEART DISEASE

As in all aspects of psychosocial functioning, a proper assessment is essential for determining how best to proceed with counseling and guidance. This is particularly true with regard to sexual functioning, given that the issue may have arisen before the onset of CHD and the likelihood that frank discussion with the cardiologist may have been avoided. In moving forward with a proper assessment, a number of prerequisites are paramount, given the sensitivity of the issue for many patients. In particular, the assessment must be conducted in what for the patient and partner is a safe environment. Privacy is essential, and interruptions (e.g., by beepers or phone calls) should be avoided. Permission to engage in a discussion concerning sexual functioning should be requested, and the patient and partner should be assured of full confidentiality. Although confidentiality in discussions between provider and patient is a requisite underpinning of trust, making a specific point of this before undertaking discussions of a sexual nature enhances the sense of safety and can thereby facilitate more frank discussions.

The language use in discussions of sexual behavior is also important to consider. It is important to strike a balance between vague (e.g., "Have you been able to return to the same functioning in the home as before your cardiac event") and overly medicalized language (e.g., "Are you able to achieve and maintain an erection sufficient for penetration"). It is also important to attend to the language used by patients and their partners because it indicates their level of comfort in the discussion. As in many matters related to psychosocial care, it is helpful to match the language of the patient, using that as an opportunity to educate and provide guidance, at least initially. It can be helpful for psychologists engaging with the patient to have specific words they are comfortable with using to describe sexual organs, the function of these organs, and the range of sexual behavior. Furthermore, in transitioning from the words used by the patient and partner and this set of words, it is important to frequently check to ensure that everyone is "on the same page" in understanding the details of the discussion.

When initiating discussions concerning sexual functioning among patients and their partners, several approaches can be effective. For example, beginning with more general questions about recovery after an acute event or hospitalization or about how CHD has affected the patient's life and life quality can lead to general questions about sexual concerns before moving to more sensitive aspects of sexual functioning. The person doing the assessment can refer more generally to other patients by stating, "Many patients who experience CHD or a cardiac event find that they, or their partners, have concerns about resuming sexual activity. What about you (and your partner)? What concerns do you have?" This normalizes any concerns the patient (and partner) might have and can "grant permission" to discuss these issues and concerns. It also allows patients to indicate either that they are not sexually active, that they have no concerns, or even that they previously had concerns but that this is no longer the case. The person conducting the assessment can furthermore directly speak to any reticence or difficulty the patient (and partner) has in speaking about sexual concerns, again by normalizing the discussion (e.g., "For some patients it is not easy to talk about sexual matters, yet for a person recovering from heart problems, it can be an important part of recovery. Is it OK to ask you [and your partner] a few questions about your experience and any concerns you might have?").

Because sexual activity is exertional (i.e., it causes an increase in heart rate and overall myocardial oxygen demand), talking about safe levels of physical activity can also provide a context for discussions about sexual activity. After discussing recommended physical activity and ways of self-monitoring for exertion and symptoms during physical activity, the discussion can move to sexual activity as one specific form of physical activity that could raise some concern for the patient (and partner). Similarly, any discussion about medications provides an opportunity to ask patients whether they have any concerns about whether the medications they are taking might affect their ability to engage in sexual activity (e.g., "Some patients report having sexual problems because of beta-blockers. What have you noticed?"). Similarly, it provides an opportunity to counsel the patient about any potential untoward effects of drug interactions (e.g., between nitrates and ED medications).

The PLISSIT Model

The PLISSIT model (Annon, 1974) was developed over 40 years ago as a tool for initiating assessment concerning sexual issues with CHD patients and their partners. The acronym addresses steps for permission, limited information, specific suggestion, and intensive therapy. It has since been implemented as a stepwise model that can be used to initiate discussions about sexuality. Asking *permission* "opens the door" and allows for a discussion about sexual activity, while also implicitly granting permission for sexuality to be of concern to the patient and partner. Providing *limited information* during the assessment and subsequent interactions ensures that the patient and partner are provided with no more information than necessary to address any sexual issues they are having (e.g., explaining that the stress on the heart associated with sex is comparable to a range of regular daily activities, such as walking a mile in 20 minutes or walking up and down two flights of stairs)—the information provided is both limited and general, yet still potentially helpful in overcoming fear of sexual activity that the patients and/or partners may be having. A *specific suggestion* is given when more detailed and expert information is needed—for example, advice might concern the fatigue issues that accompany advanced heart failure and thus lead to the suggestion that patients might consider having sex in the morning or, alternatively, make sure to get extra rest during the day, so they have the energy to engage in sex later in the day or evening. Similar specific suggestions could be relevant for the patient with ICD or the patient who has undergone coronary artery bypass grafting because of the specific concerns that accompany ICD shock or the issues associated with surgical recovery. *Intensive therapy* is recommended for the patient and partner whose issues require treatment by a provider or therapist who specializes in treating patients with sexually related problems. This can include problems associated with the issues surrounding the development of the sexual difficulty, emotional reactions to having these difficulties, psychiatric history, past sexual abuse, and experiences associated with illness, hospitalization, and drug and alcohol use.

Questionnaires

Several self-report questionnaires have been developed for use in clinical trials, and these can be used with both male and female patients.

The Sexual Activity subscale of the Psychosocial Adjustment to Illness Scale (Derogatis, 1986) has been used in several studies of CHD patients (Jaarsma et al., 1996; Westlake, Dracup, Walden, & Fonarow, 1999). It is a reliable and valid instrument consisting of six questions (e.g., "When some people become ill, they report a loss of interest in sexual activities; have you experienced a reduction of sexual interest since your illness?"[1]). Each question is answered on a 4-point scale indicating the degree of effect from *none* (0) to *significant* (3). The items, in particular, focus on changes in the quality of sexual relations due to the current illness or treatment. A total score ranges from 0 to 18, with low scores indicating little effect of illness and high scores indicating a greater effect of illness. This scale can be used with both men and women.

The Multidimensional Sexual Self-Concept Questionnaire (Snell, 1998) is 100-item self-report questionnaire with 20 subscales of five items each. Relevant subscales for the recovering CHD patient include sexual-anxiety (i.e., the tendency to feel tension, discomfort, and anxiety about the sexual aspects of one's life), sexual self-efficacy (i.e., the belief that one can deal effectively with the sexual aspects of oneself), sexual-motivation (i.e., the motivation and desire to be involved in a sexual relationship), sexual problem management (i.e., the tendency to believe that one has the capacity and skills to effectively manage and handle any sexual problems that one might develop), sexual-satisfaction (i.e., the tendency to be highly satisfied with the sexual aspects of one's life), fear-of-sex (i.e., fear of engaging in sexual relations), and sexual-depression (i.e., the experience of sadness, unhappiness, and depression regarding one's sex life). Each item is endorsed by the patient along a 5-point continuum from *not at all characteristic of me* to *very characteristic of me*. The questionnaire can be used with both men and women. It has good validity and reliability and

[1] From "The Psychosocial Adjustment to Illness Scale (PAIS)," by L. R. Derogatis, 1986, *Journal of Psychosomatic Research, 30*, p. 91. Retrieved from (http://www.derogatis-tests.com/). Reprinted with permission.

has been used with cardiac populations, including patients with congestive heart failure (CHF; Steinke, Wright, Chung, & Moser, 2008).

Questionnaires for Male Patients

Questionnaires for male patients include the following that focus on ED.

The International Index of Erectile Function (Rosen et al., 2004) is a self-report questionnaire with 15-item, six-item, and five-item versions. Each item is placed in the context of the preceding 4 weeks, with specific items concerning the ability to get an erection, to maintain an erection, and to have an erection sufficient for penetration and to achieve orgasm; items concerning sexual satisfaction and enjoyment; and items concerning sexual desire and confidence. Items are endorsed along a continuum of frequency, pleasure, confidence, and so forth, according to the specific question. Total scores range from 0 to 30, classifying the patient from severe to mild ED or normal function (Ramanathan et al., 2007).

The Male Sexual Health Questionnaire (Rosen et al., 2007) is a 25-item self-report questionnaire used to assess erection, ejaculation, and satisfaction in older men. The items on the questionnaire are worded in a culturally sensitive and age-appropriate manner. This questionnaire also has demonstrated reliability and validity, though it has not yet been widely tested in cardiac populations.

Questionnaires for Female Patients

Although the problem of sexual functioning among men with CHD has received considerable attention, this issue as it relates to women with CHD has not, with only an emerging awareness. Thus, although there are standard questionnaires that have been tested with male CHD patients, the available questionnaires for women have not been tested in this way. The following questionnaires have been tested and found valid and reliable in other populations of women.

The Female Sexual Function Index (Rosen et al., 2000) is a 19-item self-report questionnaire that has been validated on clinically diagnosed samples of women with female sexual arousal disorder, female orgasmic disorder, and hypoactive sexual desire disorder. It assesses sexual function in multiple domains that include desire (two questions), arousal (four questions), lubrication (four questions), orgasm, satisfaction, and pain (three questions each). Each item refers to sexual activity within the preceding 4 weeks and is endorsed categorically along six choices (e.g., from *almost never or never* to *almost always or always*), with the first choice being *no sexual activity*. Each domain is scored, with a total score being the sum of these.

The Brief Index of Sexual Functioning in Women (Mazer, Leiblum, & Rosen, 2000) is a 22-item self-report questionnaire that assesses sexual function in seven domains, including sexual thoughts or desires (two items), arousal (two items), frequency of activity (one question), receptivity or initiation (two items), pleasure or orgasm (two items), relationship satisfaction (three items), and problems affecting sexual function (four items). The normative sample for the development of this questionnaire consisted of 225 healthy women aged 20 to 55 years, and the clinical sample consisted of 104 women with partners who reported that their sexual activity had declined or become less satisfying after surgery (bilateral oophorectomy and hysterectomy), despite using hormone replacement therapy. Questions ask about sexual activity "over the past month," and each item is endorsed along a five- or six-choice scale of increasing frequency. Each domain is scored, with a total score being the sum.

The Female Sexual Function Questionnaire (Quirk et al., 2002) is a 31-item self-report questionnaire developed for use with women who report sexual arousal disorders. The questionnaire assesses sexual function in seven domains including desire (six items), arousal-sensation (two items), arousal-lubrication (two items), arousal-cognitive (two items), enjoyment (six items), orgasm (three items), pain (three items), and partner satisfaction (two items). Questions ask about sexual activity "over the past 4 weeks," and each item is endorsed along a five-choice scale. Each domain is scored, and normative scores are provided.

The Female Sexual Distress Scale (Derogatis, Clayton, Lewis-D'Agostino, Wunderlich, & Fu, 2008) is a 12-item self-report questionnaire for assessing subjective distress associated with sexual dysfunction in women. Questions ask about sexual activity "over the past 30 days including today" and are endorsed along a 0–4 Likert scale of increasing frequency. Items address distress; guilt; unhappiness, dissatisfaction, and anger; stress or worry; and embarrassment, all regarding sexual activity and relationship satisfaction.

Daily Diaries and Event Logs

Daily diaries and event logs are brief, self-report instruments used to record sexual activity on a daily basis (diaries) or on days that sexual activity occurs (event logs). Patients report on specific aspects of sexual activity, with questions for men (e.g., "Were you able to insert your penis into your partner's vagina?" and "Did your erection last long enough to satisfactorily complete the sexual intercourse?") and women (e.g., "Were you satisfied with your arousal during intercourse?").

FOLLOW-UP AND TREATMENT

For the psychologist working with CHD patients on issues of sexual functioning, it is essential to work in concert with medical providers to ensure that any recommendations or therapeutic interventions are conducted safely. Reassurance, placing concerns in context, and providing permission and encouragement have typically been found to address many of the sexual issues that CHD patients present (see Jaarsma, Steinke, & Gianotten, 2010). Education concerning CHD, physical exertion, and safety, with some degree of problem solving (e.g., as described earlier for dealing with fatigue in CHF patients), can be extremely helpful to patients and their partners. Working in concert with a medical team regarding the effects of standard medications for ED—how they are being used and how effective they are—is also indicated, as is the need to incorporate this aspect of CHD care with concerns regarding medication adherence and whether frank mood or anxiety disorders or posttraumatic stress disorder are factoring into the sexual problems of the patient.

OUTSTANDING QUESTIONS

As noted earlier, issues of sexual function have focused largely on men, with only more recent literature focusing on women. As this research has grown, it has become apparent that women who have experienced CHD and/or an ACS event report significantly lower frequency of sexual activity and satisfaction and almost a twofold higher prevalence of the full range of sexual problems outlined in the section on questionnaire assessment. Even among those who report returning to sexual activity, the percentage with low desire or unsatisfying activity is high. Among these women, age (e.g., being postmenopausal) is also a predictor of difficulties, as is depression. Medications can also impair sexual functioning, as it does for men (see Steinke, 2010). More research is clearly needed regarding issues of sexual functioning among women with CHD so as to inform best practices for enhancing psychosocial adjustment in this patient group.

CLINICAL VIGNETTE

Mrs. Samantha Lee was a 65-year-old married woman with multiple risk factors who had experienced an ACS event while playing tennis with friends. She was now 1 month past her event, which had been treated by emergent angioplasty with drug-eluting stent. She was accompanied to her follow-up appointment with her cardiologist by her husband of 40 years. During the examination, when questioned about how she was recovering, the patient indicated that things were going well and somewhat reluctantly asked about whether sexual activity was safe. Her husband quickly stated that this was not necessary and that he was "just happy that Samantha survived." The cardiologist suggested that concerns about the resumption of sexual activity were common for both patient and spouse, and to be expected. He suggested (a) that the patient attend cardiac rehabilitation and (b) that the couple be referred to a psychologist who worked with the rehab program. The patient agreed.

On intake with the psychologist—a woman—the patient described a somewhat active sex life before ACS, though she noted that since the onset of menopause 5 years earlier, there had been a reduction in activity, concomitant with some difficulties due to vaginal dryness. The husband again indicated that this was not important to him, though the patient showed interest in how she and her husband might resume a more active sexual life together. The psychologist interviewed the husband separately, and during that time he revealed his fear of his wife having another heart attack during sex and that he would rather they not engage in sexual activity because of this. The psychologist first normalized the couple's concerns, reinforcing the cardiologist's comments. She suggested that the husband accompany his wife to cardiac rehabilitation so he could see that her heart rate could increase safely while exercising. Doing so over the following weeks enabled the husband to feel more comfortable with the idea of resuming sexual activity. The psychologist also suggested that the couple engage in sensate-focused sexual activity without intercourse over the coming weeks so that they could get comfortable with sex again. Over the course of 2 months, the couple was able to comfortably resume sexual activity (see Steinke, 2010).

SUMMARY

Sexual problems are common in patients with CHD, negatively affecting their quality of life and that of their partners. Assessment of sexual functioning in patients with CHD after an acute cardiac event or after a change in cardiac status (e.g., advanced disease, placement of ICD) must be included as a key part of overall care. The clinical psychologist working in concert with a cardiologic or medical care team can play an important role, addressing the needs and fears of the patient and partner and, through assessment, help guide the best approaches to care.

8

Social Support and the Impact of Coronary Heart Disease on the Family

Social support is intrinsically involved in the development of coronary heart disease (CHD) and in the clinical course and recovery after a cardiac event. Furthermore, with the reduced mortality associated with CHD realized in the context of advanced cardiac care and new interventional techniques (e.g., percutaneous coronary intervention with stent, transcatheter valve replacement), more people are living longer with ever advanced CHD and congestive heart failure (CHF). This produces profound effects on the patient's ability to maintain social roles or adjust to limitations while maintaining quality of life; the associated caregiving burden on the spouse can be equally profound. In this chapter, I focus on both the role of social support in incident CHD and CHD-related recovery after an acute cardiac event and on the effects of CHD for the caregiver and the family.

http://dx.doi.org/10.1037/0000070-009
Psychological Treatment of Cardiac Patients, by M. M. Burg

DEFINITIONS OF SOCIAL SUPPORT

Social support is a complex, multifaceted construct that is defined in several ways. Some research measures social support according to, for example, a person's sense of the degree to which people in his or her life are willing to offer help when needed. Alternatively, researchers have looked at social support more objectively—for example, actual instances of support. More commonly, social support describes both the structural aspects of a person's social relationships—for example, integration or membership in social networks that include family, work, religious, leisure, and/or other groups—and the functional aspects of the relationships in a person's life—for example, the provision of income, advice, or emotional support.

Structural Social Support

Structural support or *integration* describes a person's embeddedness within society. It is defined by the relations or ties to others—social networks, the behaviors the person engages in with others (e.g., visiting friends, attending religious services, participating in social groups)—and identification with and sense of social role within the network. Social networks encompass the web of social relations or ties with individuals that surround a person. In research, networks are characterized by the nature of the relationships (e.g., partner or spouse, relative, friend, coworker), the number of contacts, the frequency of contact with others, geographic proximity, and interconnectedness—ties between people within the social network, reciprocity between members in the network, and whether ties are voluntary, high in intimacy and exist across multiple contexts. Structural aspects of support address the existence and extent of an individual's social relationships but do not describe the quality of that support or the function(s) served by the relationships.

Functional Social Support

Functional support is broadly defined and includes emotional support (i.e., providing love, caring, comfort, encouragement), informational or appraisal support (i.e., providing advice, relevant information, and guidance regarding life events), instrumental support (i.e., providing help and assistance when needed), financial support (i.e., contributing to income, paying bills), and a sense of belonging (i.e., sharing and enjoying activities with others in the network). These types of functional support serve a specific purpose, but they often overlap, and their relevance to a person can vary according to ongoing life circumstances. Emotional support may be particularly important during recovery from illness such as a cardiac event, whereas instrumental support (e.g., help with things around the house, shopping, meals) may provide the necessary "buffer" that enables a person to get back on his or her feet after such an event.

Perceived Versus Received Support

Another important distinction is between perceived and received support. *Perceived support* refers to a person's appraisal and sense that ongoing support is available to him or her, as needed, should catastrophic events arise (e.g., a cardiac event), whereas *received support* describes the actual support that he or she receives. Perceived and received social support are not necessarily correlated. For example, the real quality of support received may be lower than the perceived quality of that support.

MEASURING SOCIAL SUPPORT

A number of measures have been developed to assess various components of social support and have been validated in cardiac populations. I briefly review several of these next. A more comprehensive review can be found in Cohen, Underwood, and Gottlieb (2000).

Social Network Measures

Social network measures used in research on social support and CHD include role-based measures that assess the number of social roles, participation measures that assess the frequency of social activities, and integrated measures that assess roles, frequency of contacts, and sense of community.

Cohen's Social Network Index (Cohen, Doyle, Skoner, Rabin, & Gwaltney, 1997) assesses social networks in 12 different types of relationships, including spouse, parents, parents-in-law, children, other close relatives, neighbors, friends, workmates, schoolmates, fellow volunteers, members of groups without religious affiliations, and members of religious groups. Participation in a social relationship is defined as talking to a given person at least once every 2 weeks. One point is assigned for each type of relationship for a total of 12 possible points; the higher the number, the larger the social network.

The Social Participation Scale (House, Robbins, & Metzner, 1982) is used to assess participation in intimate social relationships (e.g., involvement in marital relationship, spending time with family and friends, formal involvement in organizations outside of work—clubs, religious institutions, etc.), social leisure activities (e.g., going to the movies), and solitary leisure activities (e.g., watching television). Responses range from 1 (*did not do this at all in the past year* or *less than 15 minutes a day*) to 6 (*did this more than once a week* or *more than five hours a day*). Parallel items measure satisfaction with the specific activity. There are subscales for intimate social relationships, formal involvement in organizations outside of work, and social leisure activities.

Berkman's Social Network Index (Berkman & Syme, 1979) is an example of a complex social integration measure, assessing both social roles and the frequency of social participation. This index measures four types of social contacts: (a) marital status, (b) contact with friends and family, and membership in (c) religious organizations and (d) other groups. The measure assesses the number of contacts and the relative importance of these contacts across the four categories. For example, intimate contacts such as spousal relationships are given greater weight than membership in groups or religious organizations. The information is combined into a summary measure ranging from 0 to 4.

Perceived Support Measures

Measures of perceived social support assess a person's appraisal of support—that is, the combined perception of, and satisfaction with, available support.

The Interpersonal Support Evaluation List (Cohen & Hoberman, 1983; Cohen, Mermelstein, Kamarck, & Hoberman, 1985) is another instrument that measures multiple components of functional social support. The version developed for the general population (vs. college students) consists of 40 items, some of which are reverse worded and scored (e.g., "No one I know would throw a birthday party for me"). There are 10 items that address each of four domains of support: appraisal or emotional support (e.g., "When I feel lonely, there are several people I can talk to"), tangible or instrumental support (e.g., "If I needed help fixing an appliance or repairing my car, there is someone who would help me"), belonging (e.g., "I often meet or talk with family or friends"), and self-esteem support (e.g., "There is someone who takes pride in my accomplishments"). Items are endorsed along a 4-point scale from *definitely true* to *definitely false.*

The ENRICHD Social Support Instrument (ESSI; Burg et al., 2005) is a six-item unidimensional measure developed for use in the Enhancing Recovery in Coronary Heart Disease Patients (ENRICHD; Writing Committee for the ENRICHD Investigators, 2003) study, a large, multicenter trial designed to test the effects of a psychosocial intervention on recurrent cardiac events and death in myocardial infarction (MI) patients who were depressed or had low perceived social support (LPSS) at the time of their MI. The ESSI was used to determine eligibility for the trial and to measure LPSS, a key intermediate outcome of the trial. The items in the ESSI were found in previous studies to be individually predictive of MI or death in cardiac patients, with five items devoted to emotional support and the sixth concerning tangible support (Berkman, Leo-Summers, & Horwitz, 1992; Gorkin et al., 1993; Sherbourne & Stewart, 1991; Williams et al., 1992). Each item is endorsed on a 1 (*none of the time*) to 4 (*all of the time*) point scale. A score of greater than three on two or more items and a total score of greater than 18, or a score of two on two items without regard to total score, classified a patient as meeting LPSS eligibility for the trial.

Received Support Measures

The Inventory of Socially Supportive Behaviors (Barrera, Sandler, & Ramsay, 1981) is a 40-item instrument that assesses how often various forms of assistance were received during the preceding month. It includes items that focus on emotional support (e.g., "Comforted you by showing you some physical affection"), tangible aid (e.g., "Loaned or gave you something that you needed"), and guidance (e.g., "Said things that made your situation clearer and easier to understand"). Each item is endorsed along a 5-point scale from *not at all* to *about every day*. A score can be generated for each type of support, and a total score of overall support is suggested by the developers of the inventory.

In summary, a number of self-report measures are available to assess the multiple dimensions of social support. Given the diverse nature of social support, it is essential to be thoughtful when selecting an individual measure or a group of measures to ensure that the assessment is properly targeted at the question at hand.

SOCIAL SUPPORT AND CORONARY HEART DISEASE

Initially Healthy Individuals

Several large-scale, population-based studies have shown the effect of social support on the risk of CHD among initially healthy people, with samples ranging from up to 28,000 and follow-up of over 15 years. Overall, social support—whether perceived emotional support, structural support, social integration, or social network scores—is associated with a lower risk of the development of CHD, for incident MI, and for CHD-related mortality. This has been found to be true for both men and women, with the hazard ratios or relative risks ranging from 1.2 to 3.8 in relation to the absence of, or lower levels of, the measured support (see Czajkowski, Arteaga, & Burg, 2011, for a review). In one study by Berkman and Syme (1979), each type of social contact assessed by their scale predicted all-cause mortality independent of the other three types; however, the effect of intimate contacts—for example, with the spouse—were the strongest predictor.

Effects of Gender

Some early epidemiological studies found no protective effect of social support for women or found a stronger relationship in men than in women, though this may reflect issues of power related to the number of women enrolled in a given study relative to the number of men. More recent studies with better representation of women have shown that social support confers the same level of protection for women as for men, with some evidence of gender differences. For example, in the Women's Ischemia Syndrome Evaluation Study, Rutledge et al. (2004) found that women reporting higher social network scores showed a consistent pattern of lower overall coronary artery disease (CAD) risk, including lower blood glucose levels, smoking and hypertension rates, and waist-to-hip ratio. High social network scorers among these women also had less severe CAD on angiography, whereas women with low social network scores had more than twice the stroke and mortality rate over the follow-up period.

Of note, in one recent study of women followed for over 15 years that assessed close contacts and social network, low social network levels were associated with a higher MI and stroke risk, particularly among married women with low scores on close contact and social network (Gafarov, Panov, Gromova, Gagulin, & Gafarova, 2013). This may be interpreted as indicating that when some structural element that is assumed to provide social support (e.g., a marriage) does not do so, the effect is particularly strong, perhaps more so for women than for men.

Although some of the many studies that have been conducted demonstrated some aspect of the relationship between social support and CHD risk that is weaker or stronger (e.g., for women vs. men, African Americans vs. Caucasians, for different types of social activities vs. others—church attendance vs. work relationships), with few exceptions, the contribution of low support to CHD incidence and/or mortality among initially healthy individuals is consistent and strong (Czajkowski et al., 2011).

Coronary Heart Disease Patients

Several extensive literature reviews (cf. Lett et al., 2005; Mookadam & Arthur, 2004) show a similar and consistent picture for CHD patients as has been shown for initially healthy individuals: The contribution of social support to recurrent events and mortality is strong and consistent across gender, age, diagnostic group (e.g., stable CHD, postcardiac event, revascularization), and type of support. Here too, the relative risk and hazard ratios range from approximately 1.5 to 4.6, depending on the population, type of support, and length of follow-up, which has ranged from a few months to 10 years after the index cardiac event (e.g., new diagnosis, new MI, new revascularization). Several studies have found the effects of marital status on survival and recovery after a cardiac event to be of great importance. One early study (Kulik & Mahler, 1989) found that married men visited more frequently by their spouses during the hospitalization period after coronary artery bypass grafting recovered more quickly than those whose spouses visited less often, indicating the potential importance of emotional support for these men. Others have found that, regardless of marital status, access to at least one supportive relationship (e.g., having a confidant, feeling loved, not living alone) is the most important factor in a CHD patient's recovery (cf. Case, Moss, Case, McDermott, & Eberly, 1992). Social support has also been found to predict morbidity and mortality outcomes in patients with CHF, with emotional support provided by partners or spouses, in particular, being a strong predictor of hospital readmissions and mortality (Luttik, Jaarsma, Moser, Sanderman, & van Veldhuisen, 2005).

WHAT LINKS SOCIAL SUPPORT TO CORONARY HEART DISEASE?

Social support may influence CHD onset, recurrence, and mortality through several different pathways or in combination, and these pathways can include effects on behavior—smoking, diet, physical activity, adherence to medication—and physiology—alterations in cardiovascular and neuroendocrine physiology and inflammatory processes. As with the onset and prognosis literature, effects on behavior have been shown both cross-sectionally and longitudinally in several large-scale, population-based studies. Fewer contacts with friends and family is associated with a lower likelihood of ongoing follow-up visits among patients who have experienced a CHD or cardiac event and, thus, with a greater number of risk factors such as high cholesterol levels and blood pressure and poorer diet.

Lack of participation in organizational activities has been linked to smoking, inadequate fruit and vegetable consumption, not having a blood pressure or cholesterol check, and not engaging in physical activity. Patients without support are more likely to drop out of CHD treatment, and for women, support at work or in the marital relationship, as described earlier for CHD onset and progression, can be particularly important. Social support also affects medication adherence and attendance at cardiac rehabilitation programs following an acute cardiac event, with practical and tangible support being particularly important, perhaps because of the assistance this type of support brings to the filling and management of multiple medication prescriptions and to getting to medical and rehab appointments. In a meta-analysis of studies on social support and adherence to medical regimens, DiMatteo (2004) found that family cohesiveness contributed to significantly better adherence, whereas conflict was associated with significantly worse adherence.

In addition to social support's expected effects on CHD-relevant behavior, it has effects on cardiovascular and neuroendocrine function and on inflammation, which has been elegantly demonstrated in nonhuman primate models and observational studies with CHD patients. Overall, these studies have indicated that social support can buffer the effects of stress by reducing the reactivity to stressors, and this has been seen for heart rate, blood pressure, and autonomic balance—sympathetic and parasympathetic reactivity measured by circulating catecholamines and heart rate variability. In laboratory stress studies, the presence of a friend or supportive relative reduces reactivity to a stressful task, especially under conditions of heightened threat or stress or in situations involving conflict.

In a review, Uchino (2006) found that studies using reliable and sensitive measures of neuroendocrine function have consistently found social support to be related to better neuroendocrine function. Social support is also associated with lower levels of interleukin-6 (IL-6). Loucks et al. (2006), using data from Framingham, found that for men, levels of IL-6 were inversely and independently related to a Social Network Index score, though the effects were more apparent for men than for women.

EFFECTS OF SOCIAL SUPPORT INTERVENTIONS ON CORONARY HEART DISEASE

Clinical trials of interventions that target social support in at-risk CHD patients—those with low support on assessment—have not shown significant effects on CHD outcomes, and indeed, there have been some troubling results for some patient subgroups. The Ischemic Heart Disease Life Stress Monitoring Program (Frasure-Smith & Prince, 1989) showed promising results for male post-MI patients who received the intervention, with half the mortality and significantly lower cardiac recurrence compared with those not receiving the intervention, a nurse-delivered educational and supportive intervention. An expansion of this initial effort to almost 1,500 male and female post-MI patients found no such effect, and furthermore, women assigned to the intervention had higher mortality than those assigned to usual care, though this was not statistically significant (Frasure-Smith et al., 1997). A secondary analysis showed that this finding could be attributed to the effectiveness of the intervention: Those women for whom the intervention reduced distress within the first few weeks had better outcomes, whereas those for whom this was not the case had worse outcomes (Cossette, Frasure-Smith, & Lespérance, 2001).

The ENRICHD Clinical Trial (Burg & Czajkowski, 2011), in addition to post-MI patients with depression, had a focus on patients demonstrating LPSS on the ESSI. Of the 2,481 patients enrolled and randomized in the study, approximately two thirds had LPSS, with half of these also having depression. Intervention patients with LPSS received counseling sessions tailored to address their specific social support needs according to the information acquired during the initial therapy session. The intervention efforts were made by the therapists to work collaboratively with the patient to strengthen and expand network ties, encouraging patients to create new supportive relationships, and providing the skills to do so. This intervention did improve perceived social support in the treated group compared with usual care, with no effect on MI recurrence or mortality. There was a significant effect on LPSS only for patients without a partner who had moderately versus very poor social support. In a discussion of these findings, Burg et al. (2005) speculated on the effect of being married with LPSS, particularly very low support. The degree to which the therapist in ENRICHD was serving as a "supportive other" during the 6-month intervention may have been sabotaged by the clearly nonsupportive spouse, and thus efforts to engage with the larger network may not have had a chance for success. This may provide some insight into the hurdles associated with "treating" low social support, a construct that may represent the culmination of a broad context that develops over the life span, the complex and multidimensional nature of social support, and the influence of demographic factors that together, by the age associated with a cardiac event, are difficult to affect.

EFFECTS OF CORONARY HEART DISEASE ON THE CAREGIVER AND FAMILY

In the title of a paper by Fengler and Goodrich (1979), the wives of older male patients with CHD were described as "hidden patients," in part because of the stress that caregiving brings and the associated risk to physical and psychological health. These effects are not necessarily limited to female partners of male CHD patients but can also be observed for male partners of female CHD patients, can extend to other members of the family, and can become chronic problems of their own standing. The cardiac event should be viewed as a major stressor for the couple and family, and their ability to adjust is in part grounded in the quality and supportiveness of the relationship before the event. As with all major life events, a cardiac event exposes preexisting fractures in the couple and family relationship that may have been managed with a range of strategies that may no longer be tenable. Even under the best of relationship circumstances, during the acute event phase, a partner can feel a lack of control regarding hospital processes and with what is happening to his or her patient partner.

After discharge and in the subsequent weeks there are questions concerning the safe resumption of sexual activity, and more generally, how to deal with patient spouses who appear nonadherent to medical recommendations, who are not behaving like their old selves, or who may show signs of slipping into a depression. Self-blame is not uncommon, especially if warning signs were ignored or if the patient's premorbid lifestyle—diet, tobacco use, lack of physical activity—was at least in part left unchallenged or frankly supported. And there is also living with the fear of their partner's death. At least initially, there is the need for the spouse—and patient—to adapt to reassigned roles and redistribution of responsibilities, accompanied by conflicting emotions about these changes. This has been found to be particularly difficult when the spouse is male and the CHD patient female. Under these circumstances, men can be either reluctant to take on new roles or unaware of the imperative to do so.

Major advances in cardiac care have changed this picture somewhat; the expansion of emergent percutaneous intervention, the use of drug-eluting stents, and new powerful pharmacologic agents have all contributed to a more rapid postcardiac event recovery and the ability of the patient to return more quickly to prior activities of living. The flip side is the great expansion in CHF prevalence: Patients live longer with hearts that become weaker. Although the months and then years after a cardiac event can be fully lived for most, eventually it can be expected that disease will progress with growing impact on life quality and activity. Thus, the spouse and family must eventually address increasing patient limitations.

As noted in earlier chapters of this book, patients with CHF have high morbidity and mortality and poor quality of life with significant limitations. Caregivers can have a significant impact on these outcomes by ensuring that patient follow medical regimens and recommendations because adherence is a strong predictor of these outcomes. Thus, caregivers absorb an enormous burden in caring for loved ones with CHF, and there are consequences for their well-being and quality of life, along with significant financial burdens. Caregivers of patients with CHF experience significant caregiver burden, and this is directly related to the severity of the CHF and the degree of care management required—for example, in the number of medications, provider appointments, and comorbidities. A positive correlation between marital quality and CHF outcomes has been reported, as has a correlation between caregiver depression, estimated at up to 18% prevalence compared with 4% to 5% in the general population, and patient outcomes (Molloy, Johnston, & Witham, 2005). This interaction between caregiver experience and patient outcomes indicates the potential value of supportive structures for the caregiver. Empowering caregivers by involving them in patient care can help reduce the negative consequences of caregiving and increase the willingness of family members to provide support while giving them a more positive sense of caring. These findings suggest a benefit for all when including family members in the management of patients with CHF as a specific strategy in the overall care plan.

Despite best efforts, the couple of which one member has CHD and/or spousal and family caregivers may reach a point at which therapeutic intervention is warranted. Psychotherapy for couples dealing with CHD can decrease anxiety for both patient and partner and promote psychological growth and increased resilience. Couples therapy can facilitate any behavior change that is needed to improve postevent outcomes, including dietary change, smoking cessation, stress reduction, and participation in cardiac rehabilitation. Therapy of this kind can guide the caregiving spouse in how to effectively support the patient, rather than relying on ineffective strategies such as nagging. Potentially effective therapeutic strategies can involve psychoeducation, emotion-focused therapy, joint problem solving, and communication-focused therapy.

CASE VIGNETTE

Mrs. Freeman, a 49-year-old Haitian woman, had experienced an acute cardiac event On a routine follow-up visit, her cardiologist noted that she seemed to be having difficulties managing her new medication regimen, and a psychology consult was requested. She presented at the intake with her 24-year-old daughter and 2-year-old granddaughter. The psychologist conducted the initial assessment with Mrs. Freeman alone and brought her daughter and granddaughter in for the last 30 minutes of a 75-minute session. Mrs. Freeman reported that she had separated from her husband and now lived with her other daughter, age 15. She stated that she had a great deal of conflict with her husband and was under tremendous financial stress. She expressed concern about her older daughter, who was also experiencing financial stress and relational conflict with her partner.

Mrs. Freeman worked in a nursing home as a patient care assistant but had limited sick time benefits and no short-term disability. Thus, with her new medical condition, she expressed fears about both her inability to pay her rent if she took time off from her job and the risk of another cardiac event due to her high stress level. Mrs. Freeman's daughter reported that her mother was her primary source of support financially and emotionally and in a practical sense for transportation and babysitting. She recognized that her mother needed support to recuperate, but she did not know how she could be of help. Mrs. Freeman stated that she was raised not to complain and did not feel she could confide in anyone about her stressors.

The intake revealed that, beyond her difficulties with medication management, the patient had a daunting number of social support needs but also a strong sense of resilience, exemplified by her strength in leaving a 25-year emotionally abusive marriage. The psychologist suggested individual therapy to support Mrs. Freeman in adjusting to heart disease and resolving the medication, work, financial, and family issues she faced. She was encouraged to use the community supports available to her through her membership in church groups and her extended family (cf. Hunter, Goodie, Oordt, & Dobmeyer, 2017). She was also referred to community services that provided legal aid to help her file for divorce and child support. Her older daughter was referred to a community therapist to help her with the developmental issues of lessening her dependence on her mother. Mrs. Freeman struggled in therapy with difficulties in drawing boundaries on the amount of support she could provide for her older daughter, though she recognized that if she continued to deplete herself physically, emotionally, and financially, she would jeopardize her health and ability to take care of her younger daughter. The therapist was sensitive to Mrs. Freeman's cultural values—the importance of helping her family—but framed this conflict in the context of the patient's recent cardiac event (cf. Hays, 2016, pp. 277–279). A referral for family therapy was discussed, but Mrs. Freeman felt it was not feasible.

This case illustrates the complexities of assessing a patient's preexisting social context and needs, which are often beyond the scope of the type of therapy delivered in a health care setting. By taking a broad view in conceptualizing Mrs. Freeman's psychosocial needs and making use of community referrals, psychological care was delivered in a holistic and coordinated manner.

SUMMARY

The disconnect between the studies showing the importance of social support to CHD onset and prognosis and the failure of social support interventions to affect these outcomes demonstrates the complexity of social support. Social support has many facets, each of which may have distinct contributions to health outcomes depending on culture and a given person's context. Moreover, social support may represent a broader and more varied concept for women than for men; at least what defines social support and how it is expressed may vary. Studies of individuals with existing CHD suggest that functional support, especially emotional support, may be the most critical feature of supportive relationships. Social relationships include both negative and positive aspects; caring for and about another person can produce both satisfaction and strain. That balance, and how to define and maintain it, may be an essential feature of intimate relationships and a core challenge in the development of supportive interventions. Questions concerning the content, timing, duration, intensity, and frequency are paramount. Whom to target—patients who have low perceived emotional support, those who lack tangible or instrumental support, or those who are not socially integrated—is also an important issue, as is how to better understand the factors that underlie each of these "presentations." Further research is needed to address each of these questions and to do it in a way that accounts for gender, ethnic, and socioeconomic differences among patients.

For the practicing health psychologist, it remains important to conduct a thorough assessment, and in the case of the CHD patient, including a spouse and/or family member in the process can be highly informative and critical to a good outcome. Even if the result of this evaluation is the conclusion that the spouse cannot be counted on to be supportive, the information will be critical to conceptualizing need and proceeding with treatment. Encouraging outreach to potentially supportive members of the patient's community and associated organizations may be useful and can be viewed as a corollary of the behavioral activation arm of cognitive therapy for depression. This exercise alone can help reveal the factors that have contributed to low social support, whether intrapersonal or circumstantial, and thereby bring useful points of treatment—including skills training and attention to cognitive obstacles—into greater focus.

9

Addressing End-of-Life Cardiac Care

As noted in the opening chapter of this volume, coronary heart disease (CHD) remains not only the leading cause of morbidity in the United States but also the leading cause of mortality. Although many of these deaths are sudden (i.e., sudden cardiac death is often the first sign of CHD), many more people die after CHD has become apparent—months or years after an initial cardiac event. This scenario is becoming more the norm, as emergent cardiac catheterization and revascularization, advanced in-hospital cardiac care, and the use of an ever-expanding compendium of cardioactive and related medications and implantable devices keep people alive well past any initial or subsequent cardiac events.

With the ability to keep people alive through the benefits of modern medicine has come an explosion in the number of patients with congestive heart failure (CHF) secondary to ischemic (e.g., consequent to a cardiac event) and nonischemic (e.g., consequent to hypertension)

http://dx.doi.org/10.1037/0000070-010
Psychological Treatment of Cardiac Patients, by M. M. Burg

cardiomyopathy. Further support for the CHF patient is provided through the use of implantable devices to address the arrhythmia risk that accompanies a failing ventricle and ventricular assist devices that today allow the patient to leave the hospital and maintain a degree of independence. Yet, even with—or perhaps because of—these therapies, patients and their loved ones will reach a point at which a conscious decision must be made regarding imminent mortality. In this chapter, I discuss palliative care in the context of advanced CHF and associated implantable cardioverter defibrillator (ICD) and left ventricular assist device care. I describe a palliative care model that helps the patient and family maintain quality of life during this challenging transition. Although the literature on this approach to care typically emphasizes the role of advanced practice nurses, it is easy to see that a psychologist can also be an essential member of a larger care team, contributing expertise on communication surrounding difficult issues both for the team and the patient and facilitating a determination by the patient and the family of care goals and choices throughout the process from diagnosis to end of life.

CONGESTIVE HEART FAILURE

Over five million Americans have a CHF diagnosis, and the 5-year mortality for these patients is 50% (Mozaffarian et al., 2016). Available treatments can slow the decline associated with CHF but cannot stop the gradual—or for some, rapid—decline, thereby contributing to chronicity and high degree of morbidity that accompanies the eventual fatality of CHF. Patients with CHF will live for months to years while enduring significant symptom burden.

The functional classification systems developed by the American Heart Association (AHA) and New York Heart Association (NYHA) describe discrete CHF stages by the degree of functional impairment (i.e., impairment in activities of daily living) that accompanies symptoms. AHA Stages C and D and NYHA Classes III and IV are characterized by the presence of symptoms that occur even at rest, such as dyspnea, pain, coughing and wheezing, and fatigue, along with edema and weight gain or loss, anorexia, and impaired thinking. This burden of symptoms can equal or even exceed that reported by cancer patients, and the consequences in the form of the toll taken on caregivers—both the physical and emotional toll associated with watching loved ones who were once vibrant and fully alive descend into an increasingly limited capacity for living—can be enormous.

IMPLANTABLE CARDIOVERTER DEFIBRILLATORS

The ICD has transformed the care of patients at risk of potentially fatal ventricular arrhythmias, including those who have a failing left ventricle. As noted in earlier chapters, these sophisticated devices are programmed to monitor the heart rhythm continuously; when a rhythm disturbance is discerned—according to the thresholds set for the individual patient—they first try to pace the heart back to a normal rhythm, and if that fails, shock the heart back to a normal rhythm. Although life saving, receiving an ICD shock is not without consequence because it can be painful and anxiety provoking, and it causes many ICD patients to gradually reduce their engagement with their world. Furthermore, at the end of life when ventricular failure is advanced, these devices can subject patients to a prolonged, more uncomfortable death through continued delivery of shock (Goldstein, Lampert, Bradley, Lynn, & Krumholz, 2004). With an increasing number of received shocks, some patients may reach a point at which they prefer to deactivate their ICD near the end of life, raising the need for candid conversations between patient, family, and providers.

Discussions about ICDs at the end of life—as with all end-of-life discussions—present some challenges. Patients with CHF have been found to have an overly optimistic view of their disease, expecting long survival. They can overestimate the survival benefits associated with the ICD implant and are often reluctant to deactivate their devices even for end-stage disease, though with proper information early on (e.g., as provided in any do-not-resuscitate [DNR] discussion) they can make informed decisions a priori about when deactivation should occur. ICD deactivation may also be seen by patients, family, and providers as withdrawing support. Furthermore, the difficulty in determining a more exact prognosis for cardiac patients at the end of life, even when death is near, makes the decision about when to have a discussion of ICD deactivation difficult; therefore, most discussions are found to occur in the last few days of life, with many patients receiving an ICD shock in the minutes before death. Thus, discussions early on that include a broad range of scenarios reflecting outcomes of advanced functional, cognitive, and medical illness can facilitate goal setting around desired health states, and these discussions should include tolerance for shocks and discomfort in relation to perceived benefits.

The issue of ICD deactivation has been explored in the bioethics literature, which has found that it constitutes appropriate management when the goals of care are primarily palliative (Kelley, Reid, Miller, Fins, & Lachs, 2009). There is often a greater willingness among providers to discuss DNR or advance directives with patients who have terminal or incurable disease than to discuss ICD deactivation, even though defibrillation is essentially involved in resuscitation efforts. Many providers have concerns about the legality of ICD deactivation. Thus, although DNR and advance directives discussions are the "standard of care," medical technology in the form of the ICD may have outpaced the ability, particularly for general internists and nonspecialists, to understand the ICD's impact on suffering at the end of life and to include preferences for management of these devices in DNR discussions. Many general internists and geriatricians are unaware that the shock of an ICD is painful, and many do not appreciate that the shock component of an ICD can be deactivated while leaving the pacing function intact.

A recently published Consensus Statement was issued jointly by multiple American and European associations regarding the management of ICDs at the end of life (Lampert et al., 2010). This consensus statement emphasizes the role of open and frank communication as part of the larger discussion with patient and family regarding goals of care. The notion of ICD deactivation should be placed within the context of an ongoing conversation that is initiated at the time of implant, thus mirroring recommendations about how to proceed with patients who are diagnosed with CHF.

LEFT VENTRICULAR ASSIST DEVICES

Heart transplantation is an effective therapy for a failing heart; however, the demand for donor hearts greatly exceeds the supply. Left ventricular assist devices (LVADs) have emerged as an alternative means of treating patients with end-stage CHF. Furthermore, patients who are not candidates for transplant may be candidates for destination therapy with an LVAD—receiving the LVAD as a terminal therapy rather than as a "bridge" until they can get a heart transplant. Patients who receive these devices as destination therapy have greater survival, functional status, and quality of life than patients treated medically, with 2-year survival from 58% to 74% (Swetz, Ottenberg, Freeman, & Mueller, 2011).

Destination therapy is not without risks, and these can include infection, bleeding, and stroke soon after implant. After implant, these LVAD-associated complications can also include thromboses and renal failure, along with the consequences of falls. Thus, although destination LVAD provides circulatory support, it may not help patients achieve quality of life goals. Destination therapy is also associated with psychosocial issues that are essential to consider before implant and also after implant, since they can place a strain on patients and caregivers. These include

- lack of adequate caregiver support and/or of a backup caregiving plan;
- a preexisting or current psychiatric diagnosis, which can be common in patients with advanced CHF, where the prevalence of major depression is upward of 40%;
- illiteracy or learning disability;
- financial inadequacy;
- unsafe home environment;
- lack of adequate electrical support;
- history of noncompliance with medical care; and
- active substance abuse.

End-of-life issues are not avoided with destination LVAD therapy; patients will die with the LVAD in place. Participation in the larger care scenario by palliative care consultants and teams has been suggested to improve focus on quality of life, symptom management, and end-of-life planning.

PALLIATIVE CARE

Palliative care is specialized medical care for people with serious illness that focuses on providing relief from the symptoms and stress of that illness with the goal of improving and enhancing quality of life for both the patient and the family. Care is provided by a specially trained team, often consisting of physicians, nurses, social workers, psychologists, and/or other specialists. This team partners with the patient, family members, and the larger care team (e.g., the cardiologist or specialist overseeing CHF care) to provide an extra layer of support.

Palliative care can reduce the physical and emotional stress that accompanies many serious and life-limiting illnesses, with benefits for patients and their family members, whether caregivers or observers. Most of the evidence for the benefits of palliative care comes from research with cancer patients and their loved ones. Yet, the potential benefits of palliative care for patients with CHF is implicit when one considers that, like patients with advanced and terminal cancer, those with CHF experience physical pain and emotional turmoil, repeat hospitalizations that increase in the final months to year of life, and wrenching medical decisions (e.g., regarding implantation of ventricular assist devices, turning off ICDs to prevent shocks and allow the patient to die should a ventricular arrhythmia occur, cessation of treatment). Thus, it is not surprising that there is a growing body of literature concerning palliative care for CHF patients and a growing body of evidence that this approach to care for end-stage CHF can improve quality of life significantly. Indeed, initiation of palliative care early in the course of advanced heart failure (HF) is increasingly recommended by professional groups as a core part of the overall strategy for addressing the challenges of advanced CHF care (Howlett, 2011; Jaarsma et al., 2009).

Despite these recommendations, few models of palliative care have undergone the systematic development and testing needed to develop an evidence base for how best to address the needs of patients with advanced HF and their family caregivers at the individual level. Furthermore, the development of palliative care models and the delivery of the associated care to patients who do not reside within major population centers presents unique challenges, though telehealth-based services that leverage the Internet and associated technologies are being expanded—for example, within the context of the Veterans Health Administration.

Dionne-Odom et al. (2014) used the acronym ENABLE (educate, nurture, advise before life ends) to describe a phone- and manual-based intervention that can be delivered by an advance practice palliative care nurse to patients and their primary family caregivers. The overall palliative care program is guided by a comprehensive assessment described next (P. M. Davidson, Macdonald, Newton, & Currow, 2010).

STANDARDIZED PALLIATIVE CARE ASSESSMENT

A standard palliative case assessment consists of the following steps:

1. Evaluate the patient's understanding of the illness, treatment, and prognosis.
2. Identify preferences, decision-making style, and others who should be included in decision making.
3. Explore goals of care.
4. Assess physical symptoms.
5. Assess the patient's social situation and obtain a social history.
6. Identify the patient's support system and evaluate family or relational challenges.
7. Assess the patient's psychological and emotional well-being.
8. Obtain a spiritual history.
9. Review advance care planning and identify a surrogate decision maker.
10. Document assessment and pharmacologic and nonpharmacologic recommendations.
11. Direct referrals both within and outside the palliative care team.
12. Communicate directly with the referring clinician and/or primary care clinician.
13. Develop a follow-up plan.

On the basis of the results of the assessment, a member of the team is chosen to serve as a coach to facilitate multiple sessions with the patient and with the family caregiver. These sessions focus on problem solving, symptom management, self-care, communication, care coordination and the use of local community resources, decision making, advance care planning, and life review and creating legacy. These formal sessions are followed by monthly follow-up calls to reinforce the training and provide further coaching according to need.

Palliative care with CHF patients and family caregivers is not without challenges. As described by Dionne-Odom et al. (2014), these challenges include barriers to initiating palliative care, triggers for initiating palliative care, and positive and negative elements of palliative care. Barriers include difficulty in predicting prognosis, making it a challenge to engage patients and family caregivers in conversations about palliative care and its goals. Furthermore, some patients become emotionally upset or angry when palliative care is suggested, and there is often confusion among patients and physicians over distinctions between palliative care and hospice care. Good communication skills and a high degree of compassion are essential when introducing the idea of palliative care, providing a balance between the provision of truthful information against a candid discussion concerning end of life. This must be accomplished in a manner that does not leave the patient and family without a sense of hope or without a vision of the difference that palliative care can make.

Determining the best time to initiate a discussion about palliative care is closely linked to the challenge of predicting prognosis at any step along the CHF continuum. The triggers for these discussions can be objective (e.g., multiple hospitalizations and/or emergency department visits within a short time span), subjective (e.g., a sense on the part of the care team that "the patient is getting tired"), or based on a desire by the CHF care team for an additional assessment by providers who focus on palliative care to guide symptom management. Emerging from these concerns is a growing consensus that the notion of palliative care should be introduced when CHF is diagnosed and then periodically at follow-up appointments, thereby normalizing this aspect of care within the larger treatment model and avoiding any shock to, or misunderstandings by, patient and family overall. Highlighting the support that palliative care offers to family members who are providing care is also important in each discussion. Thus, although they are not the same as the frank end-of-life discussions and cessation of treatment that accompany hospice care, palliative care can be viewed as a part of the larger caregiving that can make a difference for patients as their impairments and CHF symptoms increase and become more difficult to manage.

CLINICAL VIGNETTE

Mrs. Alvarez was a 68-year-old widowed patient who had experienced her first acute coronary syndrome event at age 60. It was a large event, leaving her ejection fraction below 35% and thus necessitating an ICD implant. Although she had done well in the intervening years, the past year had seen her admitted to hospital on three occasions because of symptoms of CHF. Her ICD, which had largely managed her arrhythmias through antitachycardic pacing, had fired in the prior month, reflecting her worsening symptoms and prognosis. The treatment team noted that the patient appeared tired and somewhat depressed, while also noting that her daughter—who accompanied Mrs. Alvarez to each medical appointment—was imploring her mother to "listen to your doctors" and "take better care of yourself." A consult was requested with the psychologist on the palliative care team.

At intake, Mrs. Alvarez described being tired of fighting and concurrently afraid of further ICD shocks. Her daughter became tearful during this period and subsequently voiced her fear of "losing my mother." The psychologist facilitated a frank discussion between mother and daughter in which each could describe her fears and goals and what was important while coming to terms with Mrs. Alvarez's disease status. Involvement with the nurse manager was also essential because this individual was able to frankly yet supportively talk about the clear end-of-life issues the patient and her family were facing. Over the course of 2 months, supportive therapy focused on life review, incorporating Mrs. Alvarez's spiritual beliefs (she was a devout Catholic) in decision making, and setting a threshold for "turning off" her ICD. Goals for care were established to allow her to remain at home throughout, and a schedule of daily enjoyable activities and visits with loved ones within the context of her energy level was initiated. At her death 6 months later, her daughter thanked the team for allowing Mrs. Alvarez to spend this time more meaningfully with her mother.

SUMMARY

Although advanced cardiologic care and the development of implantable devices have significantly improved survival in patients with CHD, one consequence is the increasing numbers of people living with advanced heart disease and thus eventually facing end-of-life decisions. It is the nature of cardiologic care—with a focus on keeping the patient alive—that may in part make the issues surrounding end-of-life care more difficult for the physician and the larger team that has cared for the patient over what are often extended periods of time. The psychologist working in the context of cardiologic care can play an important and appreciated role in helping patients, their family members, and the care team navigate this part of care, by facilitating difficult yet important discussions and helping to empower patients to make decisions regarding how their final days might be spent.

THREE

FUTURE DIRECTIONS

10

Integrating Psychological and Medical Aspects of Cardiac Care

"As population level data have consistently shown, 40% of chronic disease burden is attributable to behavioral and psychosocial factors" (World Health Organization, 2010); this has become a mantra of mine over the past several years. The evidence has been demonstrated in studies conducted both nationally and internationally. This volume has specifically focused on one facet of chronic disease: diseases of the heart. The role of behavioral lifestyle—smoking and physical activity in particular—has been a part of heart disease risk algorithms for decades. The importance of additional factors (e.g., diet, weight) as contributors specifically to hypertension and diabetes, both major heart disease risk factors, has also been known for decades. Likewise, the contribution of factors such as depression and stress to incident heart disease and prognosis is also well known. As described in other chapters of this book, there have been a number of promising, small clinical trials directed at these behavioral

http://dx.doi.org/10.1037/0000070-011
Psychological Treatment of Cardiac Patients, by M. M. Burg

and psychosocial risks, and thus, one might assume that with the high cost of advanced cardiac care, there would be a greater emphasis on funding for primary and secondary prevention trials to determine safety, efficacy, and effectiveness. This, however, with few outliers, is not and has not been the case.

Instead, there is an almost total lack of integration between the psychosocial and the medical sectors in the prevention, treatment, and management of heart disease. Rarely are the behavioral and psychosocial needs of the patient attended to concurrent with the patient's cardiac needs. Indeed, even the provision and implementation of cardiac rehabilitation services is the exception rather than the rule, with the great majority of providers not referring patients to—or having referral sources for—cardiac rehabilitation. In addition, even when referred, most patients fail to follow through, in part due to costs in time and money. The belief after a cardiac event with emergent angioplasty and stent is that patients are "good as new" and can get back to their "normal life" after a few weeks of "taking it easy." "Just make sure to take your medications and you'll be fine." This is the wrong message to send if health care providers are concerned with the "whole patient" and not just his or her physiology.

Many forces underlie this state of affairs, which is in part a consequence of Western thought as exemplified by Cartesian dualism: that the "immaterial mind" and the material body are separate. Furthermore, a large driver of this failure is the incentive system associated with fee-for-service health care. The marginalization of "mental health services" within health insurance policies has been partly addressed through mandates, yet the reimbursement algorithms keep access limited, especially when cardiac health care remains fractured. Furthermore, within a fee-for-service reimbursement system there are clear economic incentives for the development of new pharmacologic agents and medical devices, and these incentives drive an industrial agenda. The economic incentives associated with psychosocial and behavioral focused care to the cardiac or at-risk patient are not so apparent and are certainly not immediate—that is, any benefits to outcomes and health care use occur cumulatively, months and years later. Thus, funding for the clinical trials needed to test behavioral and psychosocial interventions for cardiac patients and thereby develop the needed evidence base must come from the public sector, and with few exceptions, this funding has been spare.

The messages delivered by the fee-for-service system are also to blame. Although cardiac patients can understand that the cardiac care they receive is "essential" and thus worthy of the associated "co-pay," they often cannot fully appreciate that any care delivered by a mental health provider (e.g., for depression and/or difficulties making important lifestyle changes) can be equally essential and worthy of any co-pay. Whose responsibility is it to deliver this message? In the current context of care that is driven by the physician and cardiologist specifically and the medical community more generally, it must be the job of that physician and that community. Yet, this community of care is largely unfamiliar with these needs and the role that the community can play in optimizing outcomes through the use of behavioral and psychosocial providers. This is a failure of the medical educational system through which future providers are trained. If the health care system does not provide examples of integrated care at the major medical centers that serve as the training institutions for future physicians and cardiologists, we cannot fault these individuals when as providers they fail to integrate a behavioral and psychosocial element into the care of their patients.

With the sequestration of mental health care in the context of cardiac illness and the overall fracturing of care, serious psychosocial and behavioral issues that weigh directly on heart disease and prognosis remain unassessed and untreated. A current best-case scenario is the cardiologist who counsels on the need to stop smoking, increase physical activity, manage salt and caloric intake, and take one's medicines. There is no formal assessment, no assistance or treatment offered, and little follow-up. Clearly, there is a need for a more integrated approach to cardiologic care, and there are a number of forces at work that may help bring this about.

There is a growing appreciation that the predominant clinical model of care for coronary heart disease (CHD), which is based on the flow-limiting plaque or obstruction in a coronary artery and the opening up of that obstruction through angioplasty or bypassing of that obstruction through surgery, does not address a large proportion of patients who have symptoms of CHD (e.g., chest pain) but do not have a flow-limiting plaque. This is particularly the case for women. Furthermore, research has consistently shown that when a "culprit" lesion or blockage is opened through angioplasty, the outcomes are not necessarily improved (Abbate, Biondi-Zoccai, Agostoni, Lipinski, & Vetrovec, 2007). A large percentage of patients have new anginal symptoms 6 months later, and there are no mortality benefits (Abbate et al., 2007). When atherosclerosis is considered as a systemic and progressive disease, it becomes easy to understand these findings. Thus, the cardiology community is coming to see that ischemic heart disease is not necessarily the same as obstructive coronary disease, and new approaches are needed to address this issue. The provider who brings an understanding of and specialty training in cardiovascular behavioral medicine, along with the requisite knowledge base in cardiovascular (psycho)physiology and heart disease, will likely have something to offer. In particular, there have been promising clinical trials showing effects for depression treatment (cf. K. W. Davidson et al., 2010, 2013) and stress management (cf. Blumenthal et al., 2002, 2016; Orth-Gomér et al., 2009). This group of specialists also brings expertise in facilitating health risk behavior change, and this effort may be particularly relevant given our understanding of how these behavioral factors can affect CHD progression and outcomes.

In addition to this growing understanding regarding CHD is the appreciation that new approaches are needed for the care of patients with congestive heart failure (CHF). Little has been shown to improve outcomes and reduce costs (e.g., by reducing rehospitalizations) for this growing group of patients. Yet, approaches that have been tested have not incorporated the type of focus and care that mental health providers can offer. Thus, this area is also ripe for contributions from practitioners with expertise in behavior and emotion because factors such as medication adherence, physical activity, and depression weigh heavily as contributors to outcomes for patients with CHF.

The Affordable Care Act (ACA) set in motion efforts to affect the equation of care. Although at this writing the future of the ACA is threatened and the articulated replacement undoes much that was set in motion, the

ACA initiated a number of changes that had gained momentum. Among these changes is a focus on outcomes as part of the reimbursement equation. To the extent this focus takes hold, there will be expanding opportunities for providers who can demonstrate that their focus (e.g., on health risk behavior and psychosocial factors) can reduce health care costs. The person with expertise in cardiovascular behavioral medicine can leverage these opportunities because a focus on improving the risk profile through attention to lifestyle and related psychosocial factors should "pay off" with overall reduced use, especially for high-cost procedures. A note of caution is needed because the evidence base on which one "hangs one's hat" has yet to be fully developed. Yet an evolution related to the ACA—the notion of the learning health care system—is taking hold. This notion includes the conduct of *implementation research*, an approach that focuses on how best to implement new, yet grounded, health care initiatives in real clinical settings and test the effect of this implementation on patient outcomes and health care practices (e.g., costs). Thus, as a complement to the controlled Phase II (preliminary testing) and Phase III clinical trials that establish an evidence base, this is an initiative by which promising approaches at a systems level can be tested, and thereby the impact on patients, health care costs, and overall outcomes can be determined. The opportunity for cardiovascular behavioral medicine is to leverage the existing knowledge base to develop and test new models of care provision in this emerging context.

Although these emerging trends appear promising, there remains the issue of how to accomplish integrated care delivery in the cardiologic "space," as the major training programs in cardiology do not train their future leaders in that area. Without this training, it will be difficult to develop and test the models needed. One promising development of the past 5 years can be seen in an approach taken by the Veterans Health Administration (VHA) in the primary care arena. The VHA has developed Centers of Excellence in Primary Care Education whose purpose is to "foster transformation of clinical education by preparing graduates of health professional programs to work in and lead patient-centered interprofessional teams that provide coordinated longitudinal care" (U.S. Department of Veterans Affairs, 2017, "Purpose," para. 1). The disciplines that participate in this program include medicine, nursing, pharmacy, nutrition, and health psychology. The objectives are to

> develop and test innovative approaches for curricula related to core competencies of patient-centered care; study the impact of new educational approaches and models on health professions education to include collaboration, cultural shifts in educational priorities, and educational and workforce outcomes within and beyond VA. (para. 2)

The educational domains include (a) Shared Decision-Making, in which care is aligned with the values, preferences, and cultural perspectives of the patient and in which curricula focus is on communication skills necessary to promote patient's self-efficacy; (b) Sustained Relationships, which promotes continuity of care, with a curriculum focus on longitudinal learning relationships; (c) Interprofessional Collaboration, in which care is team based, efficient, and coordinated, with a curriculum focus on developing trustful, collaborative relationships; and (d) Performance Improvement, in which care is designed to optimize the health of populations, with a curriculum focus on using the methodology of continuous improvement in redesigning care to achieve quality outcomes. As of this writing, these Centers of Excellence are in their fifth year, and the results to date are promising with regard to the uptake and implementation of this new model of care within the primary care context and to patient satisfaction.

How might this approach be propagated to include the cardiologic space? The vision focuses on the establishment of training programs in which future cardiologists, future health psychologists, and the trainees of associated provider disciplines are trained side by side in the delivery of integrated cardiologic care. This would provide the context for developing new models of health care delivery in which the full patient is addressed and treatment efforts are directed to each relevant aspect of the patient's presentation. The primary care training initiative established within the VHA could provide a model for the development of these training programs, using National Institutes of Health, Veterans Administration, or local funding initiatives that take advantage of local, funded internship and postdoctoral training programs in clinical health psychology. With the overarching view evidenced by the focus of this volume, one can envision that our discipline could take a leading role in this effort.

Doing so would not be without precedent. There have been—and in some cases, there remain—examples of integrated service delivery models within the cardiovascular arena. In the early days of the cardiac rehabilitation movement, there were efforts to deliver rehabilitation using an interdisciplinary model that involved health psychologists among others in assessing and then serving the whole patient. Although some centers nationwide maintain this approach, again the reimbursement models do not sufficiently support it. It is therefore incumbent on psychology to demonstrate the "added value" of integrated cardiac care: cardiovascular behavioral medicine. Doing so will require that scientist–practitioners work in ever-expanding groups to lay the important foundational structures through team science in which new approaches to care are developed and tested. The requisite research efforts within training programs and work with leadership within the American Psychological Association Society for Health Psychology (Division 38) and within the National Heart, Lung, and Blood Institute and the agencies (e.g., VHA) that fund training programs must occur. The wishes and needs of the patients with heart disease must be identified and incorporated.

Cardiac patients are partners in the development of a new model of care delivery. Behavioral cardiology must, overall, adopt and then maintain the empirical approach we were taught in our training programs and keep that focus in all we do when working with patients, with cardiologists, and within health care systems. Given the evidence that behavioral and psychosocial factors underlie and contribute to heart disease development, progression, and prognosis, we can believe that integrating within cardiologic care a focus on these aspects of the whole person will provide benefits in quality of life, "hard" patient outcomes (e.g., improved medical morbidity and mortality), and reduced health care use and cost.

References

Abbate, A., Biondi-Zoccai, G. G., Agostoni, P., Lipinski, M. J., & Vetrovec, G. W. (2007). Recurrent angina after coronary revascularization: A clinical challenge. *European Heart Journal, 28*, 1057–1065. http://dx.doi.org/10.1093/eurheartj/ehl562

Adler, N. E., Boyce, T., Chesney, M. A., Cohen, S., Folkman, S., Kahn, R. L., & Syme, S. L. (1994). Socioeconomic status and health: The challenge of the gradient. *American Psychologist, 49*, 15–24. http://dx.doi.org/10.1037/0003-066X.49.1.15

American Psychiatric Association. (2013). *Diagnostic and statistical manual of mental disorders* (5th ed.). Washington, DC: Author.

American Psychological Association. (2017a). *Ethical principles of psychologists and code of conduct* (2002, Amended June 1, 2010, and January 1, 2017). Retrieved from http://www.apa.org/ethics/code/index.aspx

American Psychological Association. (2017b). *The State–Trait Anxiety Inventory (STAI)*. Retrieved from http://www.apa.org/pi/about/publications/caregivers/practice-settings/assessment/tools/trait-state.aspx

Anda, R., Williamson, D., Jones, D., Macera, C., Eaker, E., Glassman, A., & Marks, J. (1993). Depressed affect, hopelessness, and the risk of ischemic heart disease in a cohort of U.S. adults. *Epidemiology, 4*, 285–294. http://dx.doi.org/10.1097/00001648-199307000-00003

Annon, J. S. (1974). *The behavioural treatment of sexual problems: Vol. 1. Brief therapy*. Honolulu, HI: Kapiolani Health Services.

Ayas, N. T., White, D. P., Manson, J. E., Stampfer, M. J., Speizer, F. E., Malhotra, A., & Hu, F. B. (2003). A prospective study of sleep duration and coronary heart disease in women. *Archives of Internal Medicine, 163*, 205–209. http://dx.doi.org/10.1001/archinte.163.2.205

Balfour, P. C., Jr., Ruiz, J. M., Talavera, G. A., Allison, M. A., & Rodriguez, C. J. (2016). Cardiovascular disease in Hispanics/Latinos in the United States. *Journal of Latina/o Psychology, 4*, 98–113. http://dx.doi.org/10.1037/lat0000056

Barrera, M., Jr., Sandler, I. N., & Ramsay, T. B. (1981). Preliminary development of a scale of social support: Studies of college students. *American Journal of Community Psychology, 9*, 435–447. http://dx.doi.org/10.1007/BF00918174

Baumeister, H., Hutter, N., & Bengel, J. (2011). Psychological and pharmacological interventions for depression in patients with coronary artery disease. *Cochrane Database of Systematic Reviews, 9*, CD008012.

Beck, A. T., Epstein, N., Brown, G., & Steer, R. A. (1988). An inventory for measuring clinical anxiety: Psychometric properties. *Journal of Consulting and Clinical Psychology, 56*, 893–897. http://dx.doi.org/10.1037/0022-006X.56.6.893

Beck, A. T., Steer, R. A., & Brown, G. K. (1996). *Beck Depression Inventory: Second edition (BDI–II)*. San Antonio, TX: Harcourt Brace.

Beck, J. S. (1995). *Cognitive therapy: Basics and beyond*. New York, NY: Guilford Press.

Berkman, L. F., Leo-Summers, L., & Horwitz, R. I. (1992). Emotional support and survival after myocardial infarction: A prospective, population-based study of the elderly. *Annals of Internal Medicine, 117*, 1003–1009. http://dx.doi.org/10.7326/0003-4819-117-12-1003

Berkman, L. F., & Syme, S. L. (1979). Social networks, host resistance, and mortality: A nine-year follow-up study of Alameda County residents. *American Journal of Epidemiology, 109*, 186–204. http://dx.doi.org/10.1093/oxfordjournals.aje.a112674

Biondi-Zoccai, G. G., Lotrionte, M., Agostoni, P., Abbate, A., Fusaro, M., Burzotta, F., . . . Sangiorgi, G. (2006). A systematic review and meta-analysis on the hazards of discontinuing or not adhering to aspirin among 50,279 patients at risk for coronary artery disease. *European Heart Journal, 27*, 2667–2674. http://dx.doi.org/10.1093/eurheartj/ehl334

Blumenthal, J. A., Babyak, M., Wei, J., O'Connor, C., Waugh, R., Eisenstein, E., . . . Reed, G. (2002). Usefulness of psychosocial treatment of mental stress-induced myocardial ischemia in men. *The American Journal of Cardiology, 89*, 164–168. http://dx.doi.org/10.1016/S0002-9149(01)02194-4

Blumenthal, J. A., Sherwood, A., Smith, P. J., Watkins, L., Mabe, S., Kraus, W. E., . . . Hinderliter, A. (2016). Enhancing cardiac rehabilitation with stress management training: A randomized, clinical efficacy trial. *Circulation, 133*, 1341–1350. http://dx.doi.org/10.1161/CIRCULATIONAHA.115.018926

Burg, M. M., Barefoot, J., Berkman, L., Catellier, D. J., Czajkowski, S., Saab, P., . . . Taylor, C. B. (2005). Low perceived social support and post-myocardial infarction prognosis in the enhancing recovery in coronary heart disease clinical trial: The effects of treatment. *Psychosomatic Medicine*, *67*, 879–888. http://dx.doi.org/10.1097/01.psy.0000188480.61949.8c

Burg, M. M., & Czajkowski, S. (2011). The ENRICHD Clinical Trial: Lessons learned. In R. Allan & S. Scheidt (Eds.), *Heart and mind: The practice of cardiac psychology* (2nd ed., pp. 381–400). http://dx.doi.org/10.1037/13086-019

Burg, M. M., Lespérance, F., Rieckmann, N., Clemow, L., Skotzko, C., & Davidson, K. W. (2008). Treating persistent depressive symptoms in post-ACS patients: The project COPES phase-I randomized controlled trial. *Contemporary Clinical Trials*, *29*, 231–240. http://dx.doi.org/10.1016/j.cct.2007.08.003

Burg, M. M., & Soufer, R. (2016). Post-traumatic stress disorder and cardiovascular disease. *Current Cardiology Reports*, *18*, 1–7. http://dx.doi.org/10.1007/s11886-016-0770-5

Buysse, D. J., Reynolds, C. F., III, Monk, T. H., Berman, S. R., & Kupfer, D. J. (1989). The Pittsburgh Sleep Quality Index: A new instrument for psychiatric practice and research. *Psychiatry Research*, *28*, 193–213. http://dx.doi.org/10.1016/0165-1781(89)90047-4

Cappuccio, F. P., Cooper, D., D'Elia, L., Strazzullo, P., & Miller, M. A. (2011). Sleep duration predicts cardiovascular outcomes: A systematic review and meta-analysis of prospective studies. *European Heart Journal*, *32*, 1484–1492. http://dx.doi.org/10.1093/eurheartj/ehr007

Carney, R. M., & Freedland, K. E. (2008). Depression in patients with coronary heart disease. *The American Journal of Medicine*, *121*, S20–S27. http://dx.doi.org/10.1016/j.amjmed.2008.09.010

Carney, R. M., & Freedland, K. E. (2017). Depression and coronary heart disease. *Nature Reviews Cardiology*, *14*, 145–155. http://dx.doi.org/10.1038/nrcardio.2016.181

Carney, R. M., Freedland, K. E., Rich, M. W., & Jaffe, A. S. (1995). Depression as a risk factor for cardiac events in established coronary heart disease: A review of possible mechanisms. *Annals of Behavioral Medicine*, *17*, 142–149. http://dx.doi.org/10.1007/BF02895063

Case, R. B., Moss, A. J., Case, N., McDermott, M., & Eberly, S. (1992, January 22). Living alone after myocardial infarction: Impact on prognosis. *JAMA: Journal of the American Medical Association*, *267*, 515–519. http://dx.doi.org/10.1001/jama.1992.03480040063031

Celano, C. M., & Huffman, J. C. (2011). Depression and cardiac disease: A review. *Cardiology in Review*, *19*, 130–142.

Celsus, A. C. (1971). *De medicina* (W. G. Spencer, Trans.). Cambridge, MA: Harvard University Press. (Original work published 1935)

Centers for Disease Control and Prevention. (2009, October 30). Perceived insufficient rest or sleep among adults—United States, 2008. *Morbidity and Mortality Weekly Report, 58*, 1175–1179. Retrieved from https://www.cdc.gov/mmwr/preview/mmwrhtml/mm5842a2.htm

Centers for Disease Control and Prevention. (2011, March 4). Unhealthy sleep-related behaviors—12 states, 2009. *Morbidity and Mortality Weekly Report, 60*, 233–234. Retrieved from https://www.cdc.gov/mmwr/pdf/wk/mm6008.pdf

Cohen, S., Doyle, W. J., Skoner, D. P., Rabin, B. S., & Gwaltney, J. M., Jr. (1997, June 25). Social ties and susceptibility to the common cold. *JAMA: Journal of the American Medical Association, 277*, 1940–1944. http://dx.doi.org/10.1001/jama.1997.03540480040036

Cohen, S., & Hoberman, H. M. (1983). Positive events and social supports as buffers of life change stress. *Journal of Applied Social Psychology, 13*, 99–125. http://dx.doi.org/10.1111/j.1559-1816.1983.tb02325.x

Cohen, S., Mermelstein, R., Kamarck, T., & Hoberman, H. M. (1985). Measuring the functional components of social support. In I. G. Sarason & B. R. Sarason (Eds.), *Social support: Theory, research and applications* (pp. 73–94). http://dx.doi.org/10.1007/978-94-009-5115-0_5

Cohen, S., Underwood, L., & Gottlieb, B. (Eds.). (2000). *Social support measurement and intervention: A guide for health and social scientists.* http://dx.doi.org/10.1093/med:psych/9780195126709.001.0001

Cossette, S., Frasure-Smith, N., & Lespérance, F. (2001). Clinical implications of a reduction in psychological distress on cardiac prognosis in patients participating in a psychosocial intervention program. *Psychosomatic Medicine, 63*, 257–266. http://dx.doi.org/10.1097/00006842-200103000-00009

Czajkowski, S., Arteaga, S., & Burg, M. M. (2011). Social support and coronary heart disease. In R. Allan & S. Scheidt (Eds.), *Heart and mind: The practice of cardiac psychology* (2nd ed., pp. 169–195). http://dx.doi.org/10.1037/13086-007

Davidson, K. W., Bigger, J. T., Burg, M. M., Carney, R. M., Chaplin, W. F., Czajkowski, S., . . . Ye, S. (2013). Centralized, stepped, patient preference-based treatment for patients with post-acute coronary syndrome depression: CODIACS vanguard randomized controlled trial. *JAMA Internal Medicine, 173*, 997–1004. http://dx.doi.org/10.1001/jamainternmed.2013.915

Davidson, K. W., Rieckmann, N., Clemow, L., Schwartz, J. E., Shimbo, D., Medina, V., . . . Burg, M. M. (2010). Enhanced depression care for patients with acute coronary syndrome and persistent depressive symptoms: Coronary psychosocial evaluation studies randomized controlled trial. *Archives of Internal Medicine, 170*, 600–608. http://dx.doi.org/10.1001/archinternmed.2010.29

Davidson, P. M., Macdonald, P. S., Newton, P. J., & Currow, D. C. (2010). End stage heart failure patients: Palliative care in general practice. *Australian Family Physician, 39*, 916–920.

Davis, A. M., Vinci, L. M., Okwuosa, T. M., Chase, A. R., & Huang, E. S. (2007). Cardiovascular health disparities: A systematic review of health care interventions. *Medical Care Research and Review, 64*(Suppl. 5), 29S–100S. http://dx.doi.org/10.1177/1077558707305416

DeBakey, M., & Gotto, A. (1977). *The living heart.* New York, NY: Charter Books.

de Jonge, P., Honig, A., van Melle, J. P., Schene, A. H., Kuyper, A. M., Tulner, D., . . . Ormel, J. (2007). Nonresponse to treatment for depression following myocardial infarction: Association with subsequent cardiac events. *The American Journal of Psychiatry, 164*, 1371–1378. http://dx.doi.org/10.1176/appi.ajp.2007.06091492

Derogatis, L. R. (1986). The Psychosocial Adjustment to Illness Scale (PAIS). *Journal of Psychosomatic Research, 30*, 77–91. http://dx.doi.org/10.1016/0022-3999(86)90069-3

Derogatis, L., Clayton, A., Lewis-D'Agostino, D., Wunderlich, G., & Fu, Y. (2008). Validation of the Female Sexual Distress Scale–Revised for assessing distress in women with hypoactive sexual desire disorder. *Journal of Sexual Medicine, 5*, 357–364. http://dx.doi.org/10.1111/j.1743-6109.2007.00672.x

Diabetes Prevention Program Research Group. (2002). Reduction in the incidence of Type 2 diabetes with lifestyle intervention or metformin. *The New England Journal of Medicine, 346*, 393–403. http://dx.doi.org/10.1056/NEJMoa012512

DiMatteo, M. R. (2004). Social support and patient adherence to medical treatment: A meta-analysis. *Health Psychology, 23*, 207–218. http://dx.doi.org/10.1037/0278-6133.23.2.207

Dionne-Odom, J. N., Kono, A., Frost, J., Jackson, L., Ellis, D., Ahmed, A., . . . Bakitas, M. (2014). Translating and testing the ENABLE: CHF-PC concurrent palliative care model for older adults with heart failure and their family caregivers. *Journal of Palliative Medicine, 17*, 995–1004. http://dx.doi.org/10.1089/jpm.2013.0680

Edmondson, D., Richardson, S., Falzon, L., Davidson, K. W., Mills, M. A., & Neria, Y. (2012). Posttraumatic stress disorder prevalence and risk of recurrence in acute coronary syndrome patients: A meta-analytic review. *PLoS ONE, 7*(6), e38915. http://dx.doi.org/10.1371/journal.pone.0038915

Eifert, G. H., Thompson, R. N., Zvolensky, M. J., Edwards, K., Frazer, N. L., Haddad, J. W., & Davig, J. (2000). The cardiac anxiety questionnaire: Development and preliminary validity. *Behaviour Research and Therapy, 38*, 1039–1053. http://dx.doi.org/10.1016/S0005-7967(99)00132-1

Elderon, L., Smolderen, K. G., Na, B., & Whooley, M. A. (2011). Accuracy and prognostic value of American Heart Association-recommended depression screening in patients with coronary heart disease: Data from the Heart and Soul Study. *Circulation: Cardiovascular Quality and Outcomes, 4*, 533–540. http://dx.doi.org/10.1161/CIRCOUTCOMES.110.960302

Elderon, L., & Whooley, M. A. (2013). Depression and cardiovascular disease. *Progress in Cardiovascular Diseases, 55*, 511–523. http://dx.doi.org/10.1016/j.pcad.2013.03.010

Fengler, A. P., & Goodrich, N. (1979). Wives of elderly disabled men: The hidden patients. *The Gerontologist, 19*, 175–183. http://dx.doi.org/10.1093/geront/19.2.175

Fletcher, G. F., Ades, P. A., Kligfield, P., Arena, R., Balady, G. J., Bittner, V. A., . . . Williams, M. A. (2017). Exercise standards for testing and training: A scientific statement from the American Heart Association. *Circulation, 135*, 1–62. http://dx.doi.org/10.1161/CIR.0b013e31829b5b44

Frasure-Smith, N., & Lesperance, F. (2005). Reflections on depression as a cardiac risk factor. *Psychosomatic Medicine, 67*, S19–S25. http://dx.doi.org/10.1097/01.psy.0000162253.07959.db

Frasure-Smith, N., Lespérance, F., Prince, R. H., Verrier, P., Garber, R. A., Juneau, M., . . . Bourassa, M. G. (1997, August 16). Randomised trial of home-based psychosocial nursing intervention for patients recovering from myocardial infarction. *The Lancet, 350*, 473–479. http://dx.doi.org/10.1016/S0140-6736(97)02142-9

Frasure-Smith, N., & Prince, R. (1989). Long-term follow-up of the ischemic heart disease life stress monitoring program. *Psychosomatic Medicine, 51*, 485–513. http://dx.doi.org/10.1097/00006842-198909000-00002

Freedland, K. E., Carney, R. M., Rich, M. W., Steinmeyer, B. C., & Rubin, E. H. (2015). Cognitive behavior therapy for depression and self-care in heart failure patients: A randomized clinical trial. *JAMA Internal Medicine, 175*, 1773–1782. http://dx.doi.org/10.1001/jamainternmed.2015.5220

Freedland, K. E., Skala, J. A., Carney, R. M., Raczynski, J. M., Taylor, C. B., Mendes de Leon, C. F., . . . Veith, R. C. (2002). The Depression Interview and Structured Hamilton (DISH): Rationale, development, characteristics, and clinical validity. *Psychosomatic Medicine, 64*, 897–905.

Friedman, M., & Rosenman, R. H. (1974). *Type A behavior and your heart*. New York, NY: Alfred A. Knopf.

Frizelle, D. J., Lewin, B., Kaye, G., & Moniz-Cook, E. D. (2006). Development of a measure of the concerns held by people with implanted cardioverter defibrillators: The ICDC. *British Journal of Health Psychology, 11*, 293–301. http://dx.doi.org/10.1348/135910705X52264

Fuster, V., & Kelly, B. B. (Eds.). (2010). *Promoting cardiovascular health in the developing world: A critical challenge to achieve global health*. Washington, DC: National Academies Press.

Gafarov, V. V., Panov, D. O., Gromova, E. A., Gagulin, I. V., & Gafarova, A. V. (2013). The influence of social support on risk of acute cardiovascular diseases in female population aged 25–64 in Russia. *International Journal of Circumpolar Health, 72*. http://dx.doi.org/10.3402/ijch.v72i0.21210

Gallicchio, L., & Laesan, B. (2009). Sleep duration and mortality: A systematic review and meta-analysis. *Journal of Sleep Research, 18*, 148–158. http://dx.doi.org/10.1111/j.1365-2869.2008.00732.x

Glassman, A. H., O'Connor, C. M., Califf, R. M., Swedberg, K., Schwartz, P., Bigger, J. T., Jr., . . . Harrison, W. M. (2002). Sertraline treatment of major depression in patients with acute MI or unstable angina. *JAMA: Journal of the American Medical Association, 288*, 701–709. http://dx.doi.org/10.1001/jama.288.6.701

Goldstein, N. E., Lampert, R., Bradley, E., Lynn, J., & Krumholz, H. M. (2004). Management of implantable cardioverter defibrillators in end-of-life care. *Annals of Internal Medicine, 141*, 835–838. http://dx.doi.org/10.7326/0003-4819-141-11-200412070-00006

Gorkin, L., Schron, E. B., Brooks, M. M., Wiklund, I., Kellen, J., Verter, J., . . . Shumaker, S. (1993). Psychosocial predictors of mortality in the Cardiac Arrhythmia Suppression Trial-1 (CAST-1). *American Journal of Cardiology, 71*, 263–267. http://dx.doi.org/10.1016/0002-9149(93)90788-E

Hamer, M., & Molloy, G. J. (2009). Association of C-reactive protein and muscle strength in the English Longitudinal Study of Ageing. *Age, 31*, 171–177. http://dx.doi.org/10.1007/s11357-009-9097-0

Hauri, P. J. (2011). Sleep/wake lifestyle modifications: Sleep hygiene. In T. R. Barkoukis, J. K. Matheson, R. Ferber, & K. Doghramji (Eds.), *Therapy in sleep medicine* (pp. 151–160). Philadelphia, PA: Elsevier Saunders.

Hays, P. A. (2016). *Addressing cultural complexities in practice: Assessment, diagnosis, and therapy* (3rd ed.). http://dx.doi.org/10.1037/14801-000

Hedlund, J. L., & Viewig, B. W. (1979). The Hamilton Rating Scale for Depression: A comprehensive review. *Journal of Operational Psychiatry, 10*, 149–165.

Hippisley-Cox, J., Fielding, K., & Pringle, M. (1998, June 6). Depression as a risk factor for ischaemic heart disease in men: Population based case-control study. *BMJ, 316*, 1714–1719. http://dx.doi.org/10.1136/bmj.316.7146.1714

Ho, P. M., Spertus, J. A., Masoudi, F. A., Reid, K. J., Peterson, E. D., Magid, D. J., . . . Rumsfeld, J. S. (2006). Impact of medication therapy discontinuation on mortality after myocardial infarction. *Archives of Internal Medicine, 166*, 1842–1847. http://dx.doi.org/10.1001/archinte.166.17.1842

Hoevenaar-Blom, M. P., Spijkerman, A. M. W., Kromhout, D., van den Berg, J. F., & Verschuren, W. M. M. (2011). Sleep duration and sleep quality in relation to 12-year cardiovascular disease incidence: The MORGEN study. *Sleep, 34*, 1487–1492. http://dx.doi.org/10.5665/sleep.1382

House, J. S., Robbins, C., & Metzner, H. L. (1982). The association of social relationships and activities with mortality: Prospective evidence from the Tecumseh Community Health Study. *American Journal of Epidemiology, 116*, 123–140. http://dx.doi.org/10.1093/oxfordjournals.aje.a113387

Howlett, J. G. (2011). Palliative care in heart failure: Addressing the largest care gap. *Current Opinion in Cardiology, 26*, 144–148. http://dx.doi.org/10.1097/HCO.0b013e3283437468

Hunter, C. L., Goodie, J. L., Oordt, M. S., & Dobmeyer, A. C. (2017). *Integrated behavioral health in primary care: Step-by-step guidance for assessment and intervention* (2nd ed.). http://dx.doi.org/10.1037/0000017-000

Irish, L. A., Kline, C. E., Gunn, H. E., Buysse, D. J., & Hall, M. H. (2015). The role of sleep hygiene in promoting public health: A review of empirical evidence. *Sleep Medicine Reviews, 22*, 23–36. http://dx.doi.org/10.1016/j.smrv.2014.10.001

Jaarsma, T., Beattie, J. M., Ryder, M., Rutten, F. H., McDonagh, T., Mohacsi, P., . . . McMurray, J. (2009). Palliative care in heart failure: A position statement from the palliative care workshop of the Heart Failure Association of the European Society of Cardiology. *European Journal of Heart Failure, 11*, 433–443. http://dx.doi.org/10.1093/eurjhf/hfp041

Jaarsma, T., Dracup, K., Walden, J., & Stevenson, L. W. (1996). Sexual function in patients with advanced heart failure. *Heart & Lung: The Journal of Critical Care, 25*, 262–270. http://dx.doi.org/10.1016/S0147-9563(96)80061-6

Jaarsma, T., Steinke, E. E., & Gianotten, W. L. (2010). Sexual problems in cardiac patients: How to assess, when to refer. *The Journal of Cardiovascular Nursing, 25*, 159–164. http://dx.doi.org/10.1097/JCN.0b013e3181c60e7c

Jiang, W., Krishnan, R., Kuchibhatla, M., Cuffe, M. S., Martsberger, C., Arias, R. M., & O'Connor, C. M. (2011). Characteristics of depression remission and its relation with cardiovascular outcome among patients with chronic heart failure (from the SADHART-CHF Study). *The American Journal of Cardiology, 107*, 545–551. http://dx.doi.org/10.1016/j.amjcard.2010.10.013

Kaplan, R., Spittel, M., & David, D. (Eds.). (2015). *Population health: Behavioral and social science insights* (AHRQ Publication No. 15-0002). Rockville, MD: National Institutes of Health.

Kelley, A. S., Reid, M. C., Miller, D. H., Fins, J. J., & Lachs, M. S. (2009). Implantable cardioverter-defibrillator deactivation at the end of life: A physician survey. *American Heart Journal, 157*, 702–708.e1. http://dx.doi.org/10.1016/j.ahj.2008.12.011

Krantz, D. S., & Burg, M. M. (2014). Current perspective on mental stress-induced myocardial ischemia. *Psychosomatic Medicine, 76*, 168–170. http://dx.doi.org/10.1097/PSY.0000000000000054

Kuhl, E. A., Dixit, N. K., Walker, R. L., Conti, J. B., & Sears, S. F. (2006). Measurement of patient fears about implantable cardioverter defibrillator shock: An initial evaluation of the Florida Shock Anxiety Scale. *Pacing and Clinical Electrophysiology, 29*, 614–618. http://dx.doi.org/10.1111/j.1540-8159.2006.00408.x

Kulik, J. A., & Mahler, H. I. (1989). Social support and recovery from surgery. *Health Psychology, 8*, 221–238. http://dx.doi.org/10.1037/0278-6133.8.2.221

Lader, M., & Marks, I. (1973). *Clinical anxiety*. London, England: Heinemann.

Lampert, R., Hayes, D. L., Annas, G. J., Farley, M. A., Goldstein, N. E., Hamilton, R. M., . . . Zellner, R. (2010). HRS Expert Consensus Statement on the Management of Cardiovascular Implantable Electronic Devices (CIEDs) in patients nearing end of life or requesting withdrawal of therapy. *Heart Rhythm, 7*, 1008–1026. http://dx.doi.org/10.1016/j.hrthm.2010.04.033

Laugsand, L. E., Vatten, L. J., Platou, C., & Janszky, I. (2011). Insomnia and the risk of acute myocardial infarction: A population study. *Circulation, 124*, 2073–2081. http://dx.doi.org/10.1161/CIRCULATIONAHA.111.025858

Lespérance, F., Frasure-Smith, N., Koszycki, D., Laliberté, M. A., van Zyl, L. T., Baker, B., . . . Guertin, M.-C. (2007). Effects of citalopram and interpersonal psychotherapy on depression in patients with coronary artery disease: The Canadian Cardiac Randomized Evaluation of Antidepressant and Psychotherapy Efficacy (CREATE) trial. *JAMA: Journal of the American Medical Association, 297*, 367–379. http://dx.doi.org/10.1001/jama.297.4.367

Lett, H. S., Blumenthal, J. A., Babyak, M. A., Strauman, T. J., Robins, C., & Sherwood, A. (2005). Social support and coronary heart disease: Epidemiologic evidence and implications for treatment. *Psychosomatic Medicine, 67*, 869–878. http://dx.doi.org/10.1097/01.psy.0000188393.73571.0a

Libby, P. (2002). Inflammation in atherosclerosis. *Nature, 420*, 868–874. http://dx.doi.org/10.1038/nature01323

Lichtman, J. H., Bigger, J. T., Jr., Blumenthal, J. A., Frasure-Smith, N., Kaufmann, P. G., Lespérance, F., . . . Froelicher, E. S. (2008). Depression and coronary heart disease. *Circulation, 118*, 1768–1775. http://dx.doi.org/10.1161/CIRCULATIONAHA.108.190769

López-Sendó, J., Swedberg, K., McMurray, J., Tamargo, J., Maggioni, A. P., Dargie, H., . . . Pedersen, T. P. (2004). Expert consensus document on β-adrenergic receptor blockers: The Task Force on Beta-Blockers of the European Society of Cardiology. *European Heart Journal, 25*, 1341–1362. http://dx.doi.org/10.1016/j.ehj.2004.06.002

Loucks, E. B., Sullivan, L. M., D'Agostino, R. B., Sr., Larson, M. G., Berkman, L. F., & Benjamin, E. J. (2006). Social networks and inflammatory markers in the Framingham Heart Study. *Journal of Biosocial Science, 38*, 835–842. http://dx.doi.org/10.1017/S0021932005001203

Luttik, M. L., Jaarsma, T., Moser, D., Sanderman, R., & van Veldhuisen, D. J. (2005). The importance and impact of social support on outcomes in patients with heart failure: An overview of the literature. *Journal of Cardiovascular Nursing, 20*, 162–169. http://dx.doi.org/10.1097/00005082-200505000-00007

Malenka, D. J., Leavitt, B. J., Hearne, M. J., Robb, J. F., Baribeau, Y. R., Ryan, T. J., . . . O'Connor, G. T. (2005). Comparing long-term survival of patients with multivessel coronary disease after CABG or PCI: Analysis of BARI-like patients in northern New England. *Circulation, 112*, 1371–1376.

Manber, R., Edinger, J. D., Gress, J. L., San Pedro-Salcedo, M. G., Kuo, T. F., & Kalista, T. (2008). Cognitive behavioral therapy for insomnia enhances depression outcome in patients with comorbid major depressive disorder and insomnia. *Sleep, 31*, 489–495. http://dx.doi.org/10.1093/sleep/31.4.489

Mazer, N. A., Leiblum, S. R., & Rosen, R. C. (2000). The brief index of sexual functioning for women (BISF-W): A new scoring algorithm and comparison of normative and surgically menopausal populations. *Menopause, 7*, 350–363. http://dx.doi.org/10.1097/00042192-200007050-00009

Mensah, G. A., & Brown, D. W. (2007). An overview of cardiovascular disease burden in the United States. *Health Affairs, 26*, 38–48. http://dx.doi.org/10.1377/hlthaff.26.1.38

Molloy, G. J., Johnston, D. W., & Witham, M. D. (2005). Family caregiving and congestive heart failure. Review and analysis. *European Journal of Heart Failure, 7*, 592–603. http://dx.doi.org/10.1016/j.ejheart.2004.07.008

Mookadam, F., & Arthur, H. M. (2004). Social support and its relationship to morbidity and mortality after acute myocardial infarction: Systematic overview. *Archives of Internal Medicine, 164*, 1514–1518. http://dx.doi.org/10.1001/archinte.164.14.1514

Mozaffarian, D., Benjamin, E. J., Go, A. S., Arnett, D. K., Blaha, M. J., Cushman, M., . . . Turner, M. B. (2016). Heart disease and stroke statistics—2016 update. *Circulation*, 133, e38–e360. http://dx.doi.org/10.1161/CIR.0000000000000350

Orth-Gomér, K., Schneiderman, N., Wang, H. X., Walldin, C., Blom, M., & Jernberg, T. (2009). Stress reduction prolongs life in women with coronary disease: The Stockholm Women's Intervention Trial for Coronary Heart Disease (SWITCHD). *Circulation: Cardiovascular Quality and Outcomes, 2*, 25–32. http://dx.doi.org/10.1161/CIRCOUTCOMES.108.812859

Osler, W. (1910, April 9). The Lumleian lectures on angina pectoris. *The Lancet, 1*, 839–844.

Phillips, J. E., & Klein, W. M. P. (2010). Socioeconomic status and coronary heart disease risk: The role of social cognitive factors. *Social and Personality Psychology Compass*, *4*, 704–727. http://dx.doi.org/10.1111/j.1751-9004.2010.00295.x

Pozuelo, L., Tesar, G., Zhang, J., Penn, M., Franco, K., & Jiang, W. (2009). Depression and heart disease: What do we know, and where are we headed? *Cleveland Clinic Journal of Medicine*, *76*, 59–70. http://dx.doi.org/10.3949/ccjm.75a.08011

Quirk, F. H., Heiman, J. R., Rosen, R. C., Laan, E., Smith, M. D., & Boolell, M. (2002). Development of a sexual function questionnaire for clinical trials of female sexual dysfunction. *Journal of Women's Health & Gender-Based Medicine*, *11*, 277–289. http://dx.doi.org/10.1089/152460902753668475

Ramanathan, R., Mulhall, J., Rao, S., Leung, R., Martinez Salamanca, J. I., Mandhani, A., & Tewari, A. (2007). Predictive correlation between the International Index of Erectile Function (IIEF) and Sexual Health Inventory for Men (SHIM): Implications for calculating a derived SHIM for clinical use. *Journal of Sexual Medicine*, *4*, 1336–1344. http://dx.doi.org/10.1111/j.1743-6109.2007.00576.x

Redline, S., & Foody, J. (2011). Sleep disturbances: Time to join the top 10 potentially modifiable cardiovascular risk factors? *Circulation*, *124*, 2049–2051. http://dx.doi.org/10.1161/CIRCULATIONAHA.111.062190

Roest, A. M., Martens, E. J., de Jonge, P., & Denollet, J. (2010). Anxiety and risk of incident coronary heart disease: A meta-analysis. *Journal of the American College of Cardiology*, *56*, 38–46. http://dx.doi.org/10.1016/j.jacc.2010.03.034

Rollman, B. L., Belnap, B. H., LeMenager, M. S., Mazumdar, S., Houck, P. R., Counihan, P. J., . . . Reynolds, C. F., III. (2009, November 18). Telephone-delivered collaborative care for treating post-CABG depression: A randomized controlled trial. *JAMA: Journal of the American Medical Association*, *302*, 2095–2103. http://dx.doi.org/10.1001/jama.2009.1670

Rosen, R., Brown, C., Heiman, J., Leiblum, S., Meston, C., Shabsigh, R., . . . D'Agostino, R. (2000). The Female Sexual Function Index (FSFI): A multidimensional self-report instrument for the assessment of female sexual function. *Journal of Sex & Marital Therapy*, *26*, 191–208. http://dx.doi.org/10.1080/009262300278597

Rosen, R. C., Catania, J. A., Althof, S. E., Pollack, L. M., O'Leary, M., Seftel, A. D., & Coon, D. W. (2007). Development and validation of four-item version of Male Sexual Health Questionnaire to assess ejaculatory dysfunction. *Urology*, *69*, 805–809. http://dx.doi.org/10.1016/j.urology.2007.02.036

Rosen, R. C., Catania, J., Pollack, L., Althof, S., O'Leary, M., & Seftel, A. D. (2004). Male Sexual Health Questionnaire (MSHQ): Scale development and psychometric validation. *Urology*, *64*, 777–782. http://dx.doi.org/10.1016/j.urology.2004.04.056

Rosengren, A., Hawken, S., Ounpuu, S., Sliwa, K., Zubaid, M., Almahmeed, W. A., . . . Yusuf, S. (2004). Association of psychosocial risk factors with risk of acute myocardial infarction in 11119 cases and 13648 controls from 52 countries (the INTERHEART study): Case-control study. *The Lancet, 364*, 953–962. http://dx.doi.org/10.1016/S0140-6736(04)17019-0

Rugulies, R. (2002). Depression as a predictor for coronary heart disease: A review and meta-analysis. *American Journal of Preventive Medicine, 23*, 51–61. http://dx.doi.org/10.1016/S0749-3797(02)00439-7

Ruiz, J. M., Hutchinson, J. G., & Terrill, A. L. (2008). For better or for worse: Social influences on coronary heart disease risk. *Social and Personality Psychology Compass, 2*, 1400–1414. http://dx.doi.org/10.1111/j.1751-9004.2008.00108.x

Rutledge, T., Reis, S. E., Olson, M., Owens, J., Kelsey, S. F., Pepine, C. J., . . . Matthews, K. A. (2004). Social networks are associated with lower mortality rates among women with suspected coronary disease: The National Heart, Lung, and Blood Institute-Sponsored Women's Ischemia Syndrome Evaluation study. *Psychosomatic Medicine, 66*, 882–888. http://dx.doi.org/10.1097/01.psy.0000145819.94041.52

Sherbourne, C. D., & Stewart, A. L. (1991). The MOS social support survey. *Social Science & Medicine, 32*, 705–714.

Shimbo, D., Rosenberg, L. B., Chaplin, W., Zhao, S., Goldensohn, E. R., Cholankeril, M., . . . Burg, M. M. (2013). Endothelial cell activation, reduced endothelial cell reparative capacity, and impaired endothelial-dependent vasodilation after anger provocation. *International Journal of Cardiology, 167*, 1064–1065. http://dx.doi.org/10.1016/j.ijcard.2012.10.069

Siu, A. L., & U.S. Preventive Services Task Force. (2016, January 26). Screening for depression in adults: US Preventive Services Task Force recommendation statement. *JAMA: Journal of the American Medical Association, 315*, 380–387. http://dx.doi.org/10.1001/jama.2015.18392

Snell, W., Jr. (1998). The Multidimensional Sexual Self-Concept Questionnaire. In C. M. Davis, W. L. Yarber, R. Bauserman, G. E. Schreer, & S. L. Davis (Eds.), *Handbook of sexuality-related measures* (pp. 521–524). Thousand Oaks, CA: Sage.

Spielberger, C. D., Gorsuch, R. L., Lushene, R., Vagg, P. R., & Jacobs, G. A. (1983). *Manual for the State-Trait Anxiety Inventory*. Palo Alto, CA: Consulting Psychologists Press.

Spitzer, R. L., Kroenke, K., Williams, J. B., & Löwe, B. (2006). A brief measure for assessing generalized anxiety disorder: The GAD–7. *Archives of Internal Medicine, 166*, 1092–1097. http://dx.doi.org/10.1001/archinte.166.10.1092

Spitzer, R. L., Williams, J. B., Kroenke, K., Linzer, M., deGruy, F. V., III, Hahn, S. R., . . . Johnson, J. G. (1994). Utility of a new procedure for diagnosing mental disorders in primary care. The PRIME-MD 1000 study. *JAMA: Journal of the American Medical Association, 272*, 1749–1756. http://dx.doi.org/10.1001/jama.1994.03520220043029

Steinke, E. E. (2010). Sexual dysfunction in women with cardiovascular disease: What do we know? *The Journal of Cardiovascular Nursing, 25*, 151–158. http://dx.doi.org/10.1097/JCN.0b013e3181c60e63

Steinke, E. E., Wright, D. W., Chung, M. L., & Moser, D. K. (2008). Sexual self-concept, anxiety, and self-efficacy predict sexual activity in heart failure and healthy elders. *Heart & Lung: The Journal of Critical Care, 37*, 323–333. http://dx.doi.org/10.1016/j.hrtlng.2007.09.004

Strik, J. J., Denollet, J., Lousberg, R., & Honig, A. (2003). Comparing symptoms of depression and anxiety as predictors of cardiac events and increased health care consumption after myocardial infarction. *Journal of the American College of Cardiology, 42*, 1801–1807.

Sullivan, M. D., LaCroix, A. Z., Spertus, J. A., & Hecht, J. (2000). Five-year prospective study of the effects of anxiety and depression in patients with coronary artery disease. *The American Journal of Cardiology, 86*, 1135–1138, A6, A9. http://dx.doi.org/10.1016/S0002-9149(00)01174-7

Swetz, K. M., Ottenberg, A. L., Freeman, M. R., & Mueller, P. S. (2011). Palliative care and end-of-life issues in patients treated with left ventricular assist devices as destination therapy. *Current Heart Failure Reports, 8*, 212–218. http://dx.doi.org/10.1007/s11897-011-0060-x

Talbot, L. S., Maguen, S., Metzler, T. J., Schmitz, M., McCaslin, S. E., Richards, A., . . . Neylan, T. C. (2014). Cognitive behavioral therapy for insomnia in posttraumatic stress disorder: A randomized controlled trial. *Sleep, 37*, 327–341. http://dx.doi.org/10.5665/sleep.3408

Thombs, B. D., Ziegelstein, R. C., & Whooley, M. A. (2008). Optimizing detection of major depression among patients with coronary artery disease using the patient health questionnaire: Data from the heart and soul study. *Journal of General Internal Medicine, 23*, 2014–2017. http://dx.doi.org/10.1007/s11606-008-0802-y

Uchino, B. N. (2006). Social support and health: A review of physiological processes potentially underlying links to disease outcomes. *Journal of Behavioral Medicine, 29*, 377–387. http://dx.doi.org/10.1007/s10865-006-9056-5

U.S. Department of Veterans Affairs. (2017). *VA Centers of Excellence in Primary Care Education (CoEPCE)*. Retrieved from https://www.va.gov/oaa/coepce/

van Melle, J. P., De Jonge, P., Spijkerman, T. A., Tijssen, J. G. P., Ormel, J., van Veldhuisen, D. J., . . . van den Berg, M. P. (2004). Prognostic association of depression following myocardial infarction with mortality and cardiovascular events: A meta-analysis. *Psychosomatic Medicine, 66*, 814–822. http://dx.doi.org/10.1097/01.psy.0000146294.82810.9c

von Känel, R., Mills, P. J., Fainman, C., & Dimsdale, J. E. (2001). Effects of psychological stress and psychiatric disorders on blood coagulation and fibrinolysis: A biobehavioral pathway to coronary artery disease? *Psychosomatic Medicine, 63*, 531–544. http://dx.doi.org/10.1097/00006842-200107000-00003

Wannamethee, S. G., Shaper, A. G., Lennon, L., & Morris, R. W. (2005). Metabolic syndrome vs Framingham Risk Score for prediction of coronary heart disease, stroke, and Type 2 diabetes mellitus. *Archives of Internal Medicine, 165*, 2644–2650. http://dx.doi.org/10.1001/archinte.165.22.2644

Westlake, C., Dracup, K., Walden, J. A., & Fonarow, G. (1999). Sexuality of patients with advanced heart failure and their spouses or partners. *The Journal of Heart and Lung Transplantation, 18*, 1133–1138. http://dx.doi.org/10.1016/S1053-2498(99)00084-4

Whalley, B., Rees, K., Davies, P., Bennett, P., Ebrahim, S., Liu, Z., . . . Taylor, R. S. (2011). Psychological interventions for coronary heart disease. *Cochrane Database of Systematic Reviews, 8*, CD002902.

Whooley, M. A., de Jonge, P., Vittinghoff, E., Otte, C., Moos, R., Carney, R. M., . . . Browner, W. S. (2008). Depressive symptoms, health behaviors, and risk of cardiovascular events in patients with coronary heart disease. *JAMA: Journal of the American Medical Association, 300*, 2379–2388. http://dx.doi.org/10.1001/jama.2008.711

Williams, R. B., Barefoot, J. C., Califf, R. M., Haney, T. L., Saunders, W. B., Pryor, D. B., . . . Mark, D. B. (1992). Prognostic importance of social and economic resources among medically treated patients with angiographically documented coronary artery disease. *JAMA: Journal of the American Medical Association, 267*, 520–524. http://dx.doi.org/10.1001/jama.1992.03480040068032

Wittstein, I. S., Thiemann, D. R., Lima, J. A. C., Baughman, K. L., Schulman, S. P., Gerstenblith, G., . . . Champion, H. C. (2005). Neurohumoral features of myocardial stunning due to sudden emotional stress. *The New England Journal of Medicine, 352*, 539–548. http://dx.doi.org/10.1056/NEJMoa043046

World Health Organization. (2010). *Global status report on noncommunicable diseases.* Retrieved from http://apps.who.int/iris/bitstream/10665/44579/1/9789240686458_eng.pdf

Writing Committee for the ENRICHD Investigators. (2003). Effects of treating depression and low perceived social support on clinical events after myocardial infarction: The Enhancing Recovery in Coronary Heart Disease Patients (ENRICHD) Randomized Trial. *JAMA: Journal of the American Medical Association, 289*, 3106–3116. http://dx.doi.org/10.1001/jama.289.23.3106

Wulsin, L. R. (2004). Is depression a major risk factor for coronary disease? A systematic review of the epidemiologic evidence. *Harvard Review of Psychiatry, 12*, 79–93. http://dx.doi.org/10.1080/10673220490447191

Yeung, A. C., Vekshtein, V. I., Krantz, D. S., Vita, J. A., Ryan, T. J., Jr., Ganz, P., & Selwyn, A. P. (1991). The effect of atherosclerosis on the vasomotor response of coronary arteries to mental stress. *The New England Journal of Medicine, 325*, 1551–1556. http://dx.doi.org/10.1056/NEJM199111283252205

Yusuf, S., Hawken, S., Ounpuu, S., Dans, T., Avezum, A., Lanas, F., . . . Lisheng, L. (2004). Effect of potentially modifiable risk factors associated with myocardial infarction in 52 countries (the INTERHEART study): Case-control study. *The Lancet, 364*, 937–952. http://dx.doi.org/10.1016/S0140-6736(04)17018-9

Zigmond, A. S., & Snaith, R. P. (1983, June). The hospital anxiety and depression scale. *Acta Psychiatrica Scandinavica, 67*, 361–370. http://dx.doi.org/10.1111/j.1600-0447.1983.tb09716.x

Index

About the Author

Matthew M. Burg, PhD, is an associate professor of medicine in the Section of Cardiovascular Medicine and of Anesthesiology at Yale University School of Medicine. He received his doctoral training at West Virginia University and postdoctoral training at Duke University Medical School. He directs a research program in cardiovascular behavioral medicine that has had continuous funding from the Department of Veterans Affairs (VA) and the National Institutes of Health for 30 years. He is an elected fellow of the Society of Behavioral Medicine and the Academy of Behavioral Medicine Research, where he also serves on the Executive Council. He is a Founding Fellow of the Academy of Cognitive Therapy. From 1986 to 2003 he was chief of the Health Psychology section at the VA Connecticut Healthcare System, where he also directed the training internship and postdoctoral training programs in Clinical Health Psychology, both accredited by the American Psychological Association. He currently directs the Cardiovascular Behavioral Medicine Research Program and the home-based cardiac rehabilitation program at VA Connecticut. His current grant funding from the National Institutes of Health and the Department of Veterans Affairs supports research on incident cardiovascular disease risk among veterans who have served in post-9/11 conflicts and research on the pathways by which poor sleep and stress affect vascular function and hypertension risk.

Dr. Burg has published over 125 peer-reviewed articles to date in journals including *Psychosomatic Medicine, Health Psychology, Annals of*

Behavioral Medicine, Circulation, Journal of the American College of Cardiology, Molecular Medicine, Journal of Psychosomatic Research, JAMA Internal Medicine, American Heart Journal, Psychotherapy and Psychosomatics, and *Journal of Affective Disease*. He has also published invited editorials and commentaries, along with chapters, books, and reviews that concern important topics in cardiovascular behavioral medicine (https://medicine.yale.edu/intmed/people/matthew_burg-2.profile).

About the Series Editor

Ellen A. Dornelas, PhD, is the director for cancer clinical research at Hartford Healthcare Cancer Institute in Connecticut and associate professor of clinical medicine at the University of Connecticut School of Medicine. Dr. Dornelas received her degree in health psychology from Ferkauf Graduate School of Psychology, Yeshiva University, New York, NY. She has focused her career on the integration of practice and research in clinical health psychology. Dr. Dornelas is recognized for her expertise in treating people with heart disease as well as cancer. She has supervised and mentored students for over two decades. Dr. Dornelas has authored multiple books and journal articles and is a featured guest expert on APA's Psychotherapy Video Series. She is a Fellow in American Psychological Association's Division 29 (Society for the Advancement of Psychotherapy) and a practicing psychotherapist.

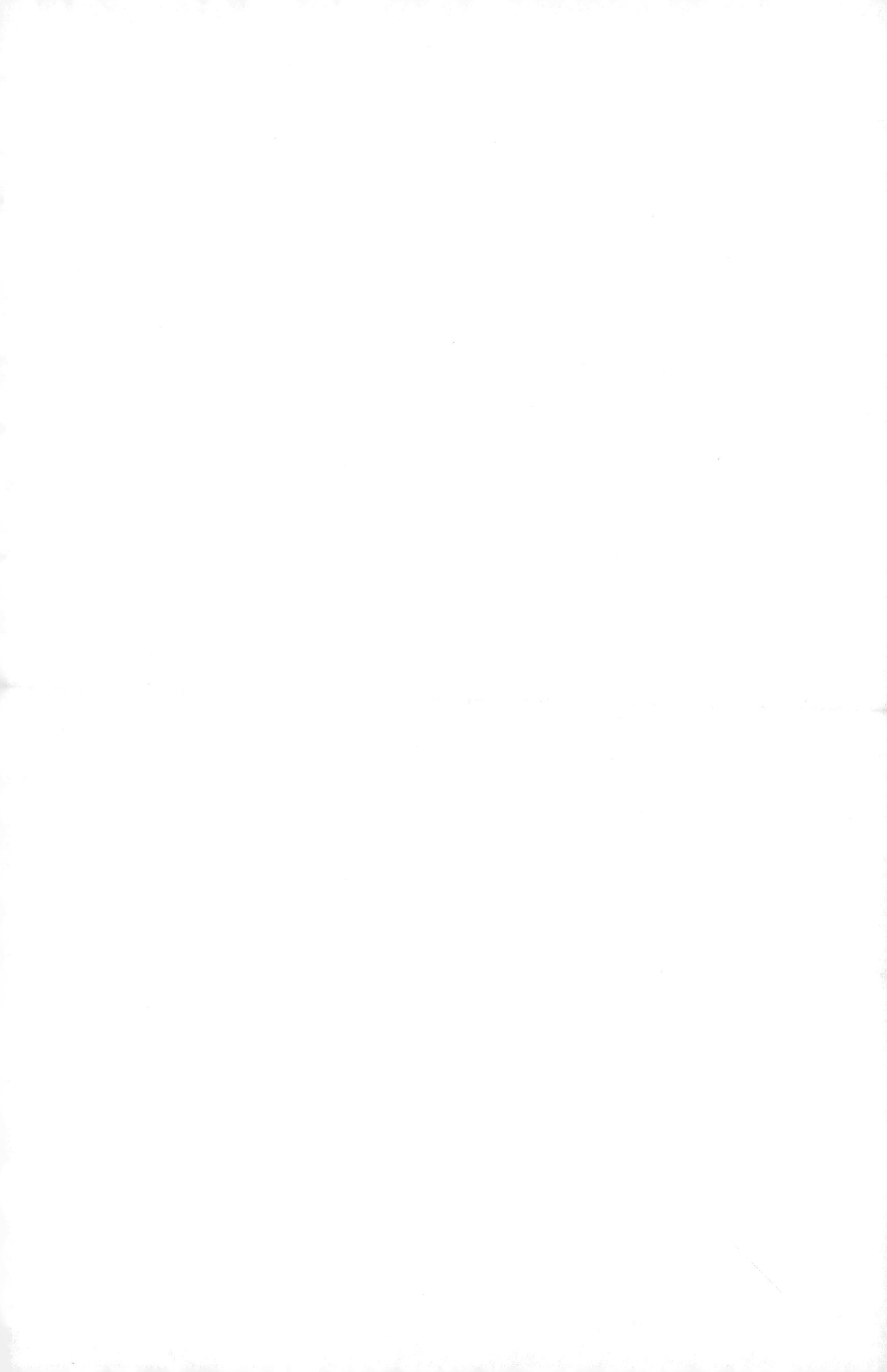